Dear Trilby

PAIN

Q & A With Dr. Milne Ongley

SIEGLINDE COE MARTENS, PHD

Sieglinde Martens

Printed in the United States of America

Edited by Kristen Corrects, Inc.

Cover art design by Natasha Brown

Formatted by Jim Giammatteo

First edition published 2019

✾ Created with Vellum

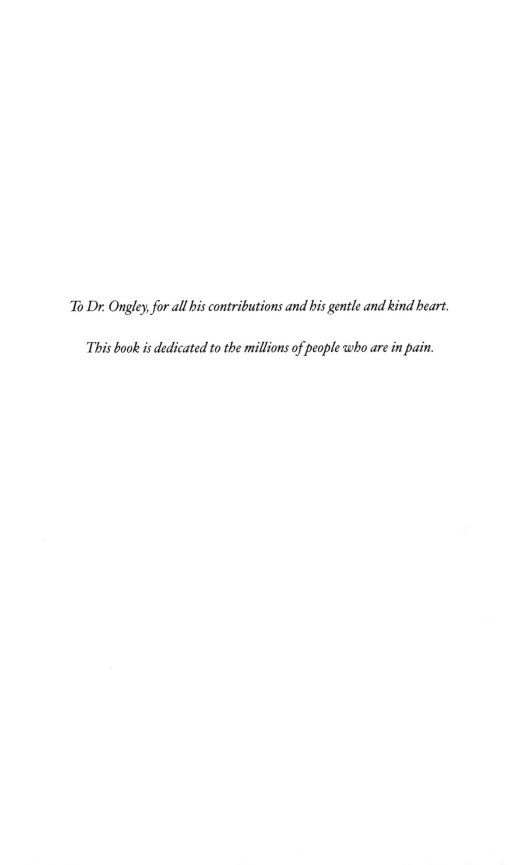

To Dr. Ongley, for all his contributions and his gentle and kind heart.

This book is dedicated to the millions of people who are in pain.

INTRODUCTION

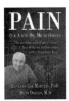

Dr. Milne J. Ongley, M.D., has practiced medicine on many continents and has cured several hundred thousands of patients in his sixty-five years of practice. He invented his own solution that is injected directly into the joints, and his orthopedic reputation is like many before their time. The greats like Tesla, Freud, Rembrandt, and Einstein also suffered being different and misunderstood—they were a threat to the established point of view at the time.

I first met Dr. Ongley at his office in Newport Beach, California, with its signed pictures on the walls of every famous athlete and Olympic champion at the time. There was an energy in the waiting room that felt soothing and loving. But the people sitting there were in pain—many in very serious pain. I noticed that, after their treatment and spending time with Dr. Ongley, every patient had a smile on his or her face when coming back through the waiting room to leave. I had never seen such a transformation. But Dr. Ongley isn't always esteemed by his colleagues. He was—and is —a threat to the medical community, which does not want cures. There's no money in cures. And thus, Dr. Ongley became a target.

Dr. Ongley may push his positive thoughts too far, but the facts are brilliant. In the early 1980s, I had four lower discs bone on bone and had problems turning over in bed and was in constant pain. I was referred to him by a friend and had one set of injections. He told me to do these very simple exercises which took no more than ten minutes, and by the third month I was already feeling great. I had an x-ray six months after treatment and the discs had grown back to their normal selves—my problem was solved. Over the years of falling and breaking parts of my skeleton, he was my doctor and became a very close and dear friend. Without him I would be in a wheelchair by now because opting for invasive surgery would never be my first choice.

I have spent much time with him over the last thirty-three years and know he is very loving but stands only in truth and integrity and what is best for the patient. He is both gentle and firm. I learned the magic of the body and how unaware we each are related to pain, be it the real cause, the location, and the message it holds for the patient. All of this led to us sitting down having a rather long chat, which led to the information in this book.

I know this will be a refreshing wake-up call for many to take responsibility for their own health without putting the medical community on a pedestal. Thoughts, emotions, and pain are the topics of focus in this book. Our multiple prescriptions give us a false sense of safety, but I consider those prescriptions a trap set by the medical community.

We live in our self-created prison...but the door is not locked. Let's walk free to live our life.

Sieglinde Coe Martens, Ph.D.

Chapter One

TREATMENT OF LOW BACK PAIN

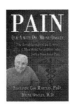

Treatment of the Low Back and Neck

Low back injuries are certainly not uncommon. Presumably this is something to which you can readily testify. Indeed, musculoskeletal pain of some body part is experienced by all of us at some time or another. The low back is particularly predisposed to such insult, resultant discomfort and overall malfunction. The nature of the insult may be well recalled in detail by the patient or, he or she may not be able to attribute the damaging incident to anything specific. Regardless of these details, the patient is in pain, probably to the degree to which daily activities which once were commonplace, and able to be performed without forethought, now require advance planning and assistance if they can even be carried out at all. Such endeavors become taxing on the patient not to mention family members and others who are investing their efforts in the assistance of the afflicted. This perhaps is a more severe scenario than that experienced by most of us who "get along" and complete our daily activities in varying degrees of discomfort and disability. At some point we may have reached the stage of seeking professional help. We may have visited a Chiropractor, Osteopathic physician,

Orthopaedic surgeon, Neurosurgeon, Deep Tissue Masseur, Physical Therapist, Acupuncturist or any of the absolutely bewildering array of practitioners claiming to have the state of the art treatment for musculoskeletal disorders such as your low back dysfunction.

Let us take a moment to look at what it is they offer, what it may do for you and, most importantly, what it is that is wrong with you. This last concept is of the utmost importance as it is absolutely essential to really understand what is wrong before a sensible and successful treatment plan can be made and carried out successfully.

Chiropractic

Folks who practice this discipline are well known by name to the typical person in today's society. They are the people who use a form of manipulation to "put you back into place". Their art is, of course, a bit more complicated than that and there are various schools of thought within the Chiropractic world. They will likely speak of "pinched nerves" and the necessity of relieving such pressure by way of manipulation. Generally speaking, this will result in a degree of relief for the patient who is now very pleased indeed to be free of the pain which was so impairing his lifestyle. Yes, nerve roots exiting the cord do so by passing through a hole in the bony part of the spinal column. These "neural foramina" are certainly altered in size and shape by vertebral subluxation (out of placeness) and this results in the "pinched nerve" condition. A Chiropractic manipulation will realign the vertebrae in question, returning the foramen to its proper dimensions thereby relieving the pressure on the "pinched nerve", and taking away the patient's pain. This all seems quite reasonable until one considers that many such patients continue to return to their Chiropractor in the future for continuing "adjustments" as the return of their old discomfort dictates. Why? Did the initial manipulation not take care of the problem? What else is wrong to necessitate repeated visits to the practitioner?

The answer comes with an understanding of the nature of the initial injury. When this is uncovered it becomes clear that realignment of the involved bony structures, while necessary, is only a temporary solution at best and, at worst, ultimately as detrimental to the patient as was the original injury.

Osteopathic medicine

Osteopathy began not too unlike Chiropractic i.e. utilizing manipulation alone as their mainstay of treatment. As time passed, they began to incorporate "mainstream" methodologies into their repertoire as the Allopaths endorsed. This, really is not much different from chiropractic, and while temporarily able to restore strength and relieve pain, still is not the answer for which we search.

Surgery

Orthopaedic and Neurological Surgery shall be discussed together as they essentially employ the same approach to the management of back and neck pain. These fields are considered to be allopathic and so fall into the mainstream of American medicine.

Typically, the approach to such ailments involves a period of watchful waiting accompanied by anti-inflammatories, muscular relaxants, pain killers, bed rest, immobilization etc.. When this invariably fails to be satisfactory, a trial of physical therapy is instituted. By now the patient has been drugged, restrained from daily activities such as employment (not to mention recreation and loss of wages). For most folks this is nothing short of frustrating in the highest. Upon the scheduled return to the allopathic M.D., a reevaluation of the patients condition will be made. Typically this will consist of a review of the most recent images (X-Ray, C.T., MRI etc.) a perfunctory exam of the actual patient will be carried out also. It should be fairly obvious to all that a person who has undergone a period of extended inactivity in conjunction with a pharmacological onslaught of pain pills and muscular relaxing agents will not only still be in pain but also now profoundly weakened despite any prescribed physical therapy.

Pain and weakness persisting in the face of the traditional conservative measures outlined above are the accepted criteria for the next "logical" step in the allopathic algorithm—Surgery!

Acupuncture

The treatment modality known as acupuncture may be effective in temporarily relieving the pain associated with the injuries described above. It is able to be effective temporarily as it does interrupt the pain reflex arc by interfering with neuronal (nerve) transmission of the painful stimuli. This, however is the extent of its capability and is by no means a treatment for the problem causing the pain and disability from which the patient suffers. So just what is this malady to which most of us, if not all, succumb at some time or another. Let us first explore what a spinal column is and how it is put

together.

A Revised Approach to Spinal Pain

The human spinal column includes the neck and the back. Within its bony armor is a bundle of nerves and nerve roots known as the spinal cord. The spinal roots which come off of the cord at various levels exit this osseous tube by way of the foramina mentioned earlier. Foramina are formed by the juncture of two vertebrae and are found one on either side of a vertebral pair. The vertebrae have a cushion between them commonly referred to as a disc. The bony vertebrae themselves are tethered one to the other by a class of connective tissue known as ligaments. Ligaments are collagenous structures which hold bones to other bones whereas tendons are the collagenous attachments of muscles to bone. When we descend the vertebral column as far as the pelvis, we find that several vertebrae have become fused into the triangular bone we now refer to as the sacrum. The sacrum is part of the pelvic girdle and articulates (forms joints) with the wing -shaped iliac bones. This is the famous sacroiliac joint we all hear so much about.

But what about the injury?

So far we have discovered that there are a lot of structures in the spine which may be injured. To sort through all of this a logical methodology based upon patterns of pain referral and functional testing has been developed so as to lead the practitioner to the correct diagnosis. Great. Now what do you do? Massage? Acupuncture? Surgery, and if so, on what? Chiropractic manipulation, and if so, on what and for how long? To clarify, if we have been accurate in our diagnosis there are only a few structures which will be involved. Let us begin with the most common, ligaments.

Ligaments, as you will recall, hold our vertebrae together. When our vertebrae

become misaligned due to some mishap, the ligaments become stretched. Until very recently it was believed that a ligament once stretched would remain so. Indeed, without appropriate intervention this would remain the case. This is why Chiropractors and Osteopaths manipulate the spine in order to reimpose appropriate mechanics to the injured area. In severe instances, the instability may be so great that repeated manipulations would be to no avail and in would step the Orthpaedic surgeon who would likely remedy this situation with a vertebral fusion. This, of course, gives the spine in question a diminished degree of flexibility. Let us assume that there was a way to cause a ligament to tighten up while retaining the normal degree of flexibility all without surgery or repeated manipulations. Would this be something that you might opt for were you to be so unfortunate as to have injured your spine? Well, let us assume no longer, for such a way exists. Now let's see what this entails.

What You Can Expect

Ok, so you've hurt your neck, or back, or both. Now you find yourself considering something you probably have not heard of before or perhaps know only a little about.

We will start with the neck.

Necks are important. We need them for everything we do.

Naturally you are likely to be apprehensive about anybody doing anything to yours. To help relax you, we administer a mild intravenous muscle relaxant to take the tension out of you in a way that you can not voluntarily do. Next we sterilize the skin on the back of the neck, and begin to infiltrate the painful soft tissues with a local anesthetic just like the type used during dental procedures. Those soft tissues are ligaments and muscles which have likely been operating under stress due to your injury. The anesthetic is introduced by a needle and is generally perceived as a "pressure" in the neck. A small amount of a synthetic corticosteroid (Triamcinolone) is also introduced. This anti-inflammatory has been carefully engineered so as to be effective yet avoid the adverse efffects associated with its chemical cousin, Cortisone. Following this injection, you will be turned over and a small amount of traction will be applied to your neck so as to realign those structures which are maligned. This may feel strange but is certainly neither painful, nor dangerous. So ends your initial neck treatment.

The initial back treatment differs very little except in that the treatment involves the low back and it is the sacrum which is manipulated. In each case, the one manipulation should be all that is required in this regard.

Day two involves the first of a series of injections into the involved ligaments.

Ideally these would be administered at weekly intervals. A minimum of six for the neck, and a minimum of eight for the back. Certainly it is possible for a patient to skip a week, or even two, although this is not recommended.

What do these injections do? For a full explanation we refer you to the pamphlet "What is a proliferant". In short, however, they are causing a controlled form of inflammation resulting in the deposition of new collagenous material in the lines of force of the ligament. This is why this treatment is not "sclerotherapy".

Alright, we have done our part. We have realigned you, and stimulated your ligaments to become shorter, thicker, stronger and develop larger areas of attachment to bone. That was the easy part. The hard part is just beginning and is totally dependent upon you. The proliferant will continue to develop your ligaments for some nine months or so. You must accept responsibility for the majority of your rehabilitation. We shall provide you with movements to be performed with religious devotion. We shall make recommendations for changes in lifestyle where we see fit but ultimately it all depends on you.

Chapter Two

QUESTIONS & ANSWERS

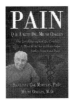

Dr. Milne J Ongley, a legend in his own time, shares sixty-five years of experience.

Dr. Ongley

If we get three thousand women together in a large meeting place and ask them the question, How many of you have back pain and have ever suffered from back pain, how many do you suppose stand up?

Sieglinde

I would imagine all of them.

Dr. Ongley

Then if you told them there is absolutely no need whatsoever to suffer from back pain now or in the future, would they believe you?

. . .

Sieglinde

Probably not.

Dr. Ongley

Then shouldn't our object be some way to figure out a way to convince all of those three thousand women that back pain is perfectly curable by explaining the causation of back pain? We are not talking about back pain caused by spinal tumors, tuberculosis, or cancer but the common variety of back pain.

Then to dispel the myth that if you are pregnant there is no scientific reason why a person who is having a baby should not have back pain or when that person has given birth to a baby it's not necessary for her while carrying or after the birth to have back pain.

This is why I have selected an audience of three thousand women because they will say, "Ha, we haven't heard of that before!" Then why is it when they are having a period they should have back pain? In medicine we are all aware that most times we feel pain. The pain is relayed by the nervous system. Generally speaking, you have to have a nerve in the area that is being traumatized or sends a message up to your brain where you feel pain. There is no nerve connecting the uterus with the back. Why on earth does the female of the species who has something happening in her uterus, not necessarily something abnormal, have back pain? Pregnancy is not an abnormal state. Why should they have this abnormality of back pain?

. . .

Sieglinde

Then why do women say they have this pain?

Dr. Ongley

That is an interesting question, isn't it? Let us take a person with a heart attack he feels pain in his neck and down the left side of his arm. There is no nerve from the heart to the arm, so how on earth does he feel the pain in his arm? Then you have the problem of the woman who has had a surgical removal of the breast and she feels pain in the breast, or an amputee who has no arm yet he or she still feels the pain in the area that is no longer a part of the physical body. So, in the human body, it is impossible to accept that pain has traveled down a nerve. Pain is transferred.

Sieglinde

So what you are saying is that the brain holds the memory of an arm or a breast even when it is removed?

Dr. Ongley

That is correct. This immediately makes the jump ahead and points out that if the patient comes in complaining of pain in the arm, in reality the problem is in the heart. It is rather pointless to direct any type of treatment to the arm. Or if someone has a pain in the back or in the lower lip, it is pointless to direct treatment to the lower lip. We must direct meaningful treatment to the site of the problem.

Sieglinde

What is meaningful treatment and how do you know the site of the problem?

. . .

Dr. Ongley

Just as the heart gives pain to a certain area of the problem, is it not reasonable to suggest that other known areas of the body will send pain to another specified area? So if you check the area where the pain is being felt by the patient, you should then know from whence it arises. The scientific knowledge for this has been around for centuries. Why do health professionals choose not to avail themselves to this knowledge? Why do we allow ourselves to be treated by the physical therapy means of heat, light, sound, et cetera, applied to the area which is not the source of pain?

Sieglinde

What makes people so vulnerable to whatever treatment is prescribed?

Dr. Ongley

If patients had this knowledge, they would not allow ultra-sonic or any other physical therapeutic means to be applied to the wrong area. Most people today who might have a pain in the abdomen expect to be treated in the abdomen and are not likely to accept treatment in the big toe. Somehow this information, which is readily available, must get out to the general public. When a patient goes to a physician for help, he doesn't treat the "wrong" part of the body.

Sieglinde

What you're saying, then, is we must each take responsibility for issues occurring in our body.

. . .

Dr. Ongley

Yes. We had talked previously about the overriding controls of the emotional centers in the brain concerning pain. Wouldn't it be nice if most people were cognizant of that fact?

Sieglinde

What is pain?

Dr. Ongley

That depends on your religious and moral upbringing. If you do wrong, the teacher will say, "I will give you pain." Pain now becomes a punishment or penalty. In fact, the word pain comes from the Latin word *poena*, which means punishment or penalty. In Old English they had a completely different word for what we'll term bodily suffering, the law, so they were two separate entities—pain, the law and bodily suffering.

Historically, King James I's edition of the true Bible confused the words. Shakespeare and Chaucer did not have two separate words with two separate meanings. In 1616 editions of the Bible confused them so that the word pain meant some circumstances of bodily suffering in others penalty or punishment. So if you are the type of person who believes you are supposed to suffer in this world, then pain for you is glorification. It gives you moral fiber.

When the area that is damaged or the site of the chemical imbalance stimulates the little pain fibers, their ultimate destination in the brain is the same area of the brain where you feel emotions. The area of the brain that you hate is where you feel pain. It's the same experience. It's not a sensation like spelling or seeing an experience. So shall we say that if in that area ninety percent of the little cells are taken up with sorrow and you add in what we understand as pain, now that unpleasant emotional experience is going to be much more severe for the patient. If he is happy, you give him the same amount of pain he is not going to feel so much of that unpleasant emotional experience.

Sieglinde

Are you saying that pain and pleasure reside in the same part of the brain and the happier we are, we have less room for pain?

Dr. Ongley

Correct. People who are emotionally unstable, when something is inflicted upon their body which normally would give X amount of pain, because of the mental state, they are now given ten times the pain and until the physicians become aware that the mental state of the patient is of paramount importance when they are controlling pain. People will suffer when they don't need to. Instead, prescriptions are the answer today, confusing and causing additional challenges in the immune system and every part of the person's body.

Sieglinde

When a doctor is treating a patient, how concerned is he about the pain?

Dr. Ongley

Generally he is very concerned about the pain but he is not concerned about the patient. The physician should have an individual approach.

. . .

There is usually a very good reason why the physician is concentrating on the pain and not the patient. For example let us suppose you're a surgeon and you are trying to figure out if the patient has appendicitis—you must concentrate on the pain to make a diagnosis; however, where the physician is skipping out is that the pain is attached to a patient, therefore treat the patient as well as the origin.

Sieglinde

Where does the physician gain the skill to treat the origin of disease?

Dr. Ongley

From the patient by listening, observing how he sits, stands, how he reacts to questions. In medical school unfortunately he is taught the external characteristics of disease unless he is in a psychiatric field. Physicians should spend more time evaluating the mental state of an individual patient. The scientific reason is that pain is an unpleasant emotional experience. Now how do you judge experience? Have you had it before, do you still have the memory of it? All of these things are contributing factors in how a doctor should approach pain in a patient.

Sieglinde

How long have you been healing people?

Dr. Ongley

A long time. Since I graduated medical school. More than sixty years.

. . .

Sieglinde

When you look at a patient what is the first thing you see?

Dr. Ongley

Since I am in the pain field, I get a pretty good clue when the patient comes in if the patient is truly suffering

severe pain, mild pain, or moderate pain. If they hop in with a compound fracture of their lower leg and they are still smiling at me, then wow, I have to ask how can this person be smiling. Someone else will come in with a thorn sticking in their skin and they will be shouting and screaming and carrying on and they are in complete agony. So there is a very marked difference of the site and the extent of the injury and the patient. How come?

Sieglinde

What causes the difference in the threshold of pain?

Dr. Ongley

Some people are able, through their perceptual experience, their memory in that area of the brain, to modulate the experience of pain. And we all know that in older days you could have a sword stuck in your ribs during battle you wouldn't even be aware of.

I'm sure if I took a sword and stuck it in your ribs here and now you would scream and holler in pain. Why is it that if I put you in a situation of fighting and defending your child's life and you received a knife in the chest, you would not be aware of it? It is because your focus is not on the pain. Mental control modulates pain.

·   ·   ·

Sieglinde

Once again, when you see a patient, what do you see?

Dr. Ongley

Most important of all, once again the patient must be put in a category through observation. Observation based on experience. Seeing what is not apparent to most people. A little like Rembrandt. He sees much more than the average person. He is able to put what he sees onto a canvas where most people will just do an outline and Rembrandt sees wondrous detail. It is the art of seeing.

Sieglinde

How are you like Rembrandt?

Dr. Ongley

I have taught myself to observe so-called body and energetic language which exudes from every living thing. This can be learned and translated. An example of this is a seventeen-year-old athletic girl walking down the street. She walks with a spring in her step as she passes. Her eyes are not bloodshot; you note she has a hue in her cheeks, a smile on her face, her teeth are even and white when she says good morning; you notice her tongue is not dirty. You don't need to be a physician to see that this girl is healthy. She walks correctly; she is observant of her surroundings. She doesn't have big lumps and bumps all over her face, clarity of eyes—her body can't be filled with toxins. Why is this such a mystery when someone transferred into a clinic makes the same observation. It's no different. It's just a matter of degree.

Sieglinde

I have observed middle-aged persons walk into your clinic, depressed, in pain, limping, sad, in agony, looking cumbersome, feeling hopelessness. Within ten minutes they come out with a bounce in their step, a smile on their face, and happy. It's as if they have a new lease on life. How do you do that each and every time?

Dr. Ongley

Hope springs eternal.

Sieglinde

That is too simple.

Dr. Ongley

Simple things are the correct things. The biggest problem in medicine today is that it has become much too complicated and the passion for healing is lost. Once you spend the time with a patient and you know what is wrong with them and you can help them with their problem and truly observe and treat them, you have done your job. People feel respected and cared for and their pain may cease to exist.

When was the last time you really observed another person carefully? Most people never notice or observe anyone. Physicians in particular do not observe enough. If they did, not only would their passion come into their work, but they would be much more successful. By being successful, it would be rewarding for not only for the patient but also for the doctor.

Sieglinde

What keeps doctors from really wanting to observe?

Dr. Ongley

That's the same question you should ask the artist and the person who is not an artist. The person with the camera, he will tell you it is in the art of seeing, he sees pictures and takes them, the things you and I don't see. So what we should do is spend much more time training the physician in the art of observing their patients and what the observations mean.

Sieglinde

Observing and what the observation means are separate issues and could be interpreted differently since everyone filters information through his personal experience.

Dr. Ongley

Therefore, in the belly just as we have pain, vomiting, and constipation, temperature, rigidity...we say that person could have appendicitis. Why can't we look at the clarity of the eyes, the skin, the tongue, and the overall mode of acceptance of that particular individual at the time and say she is happy or she is sad? If she is happy, why is she happy? If she is sad, why is she sad?

Sieglinde

So you feel a doctor should want to know these things? Might this not open a can of worms that he doesn't want to deal with or even care about, or have time for?

Dr. Ongley

This is the problem with the medical system—it is not the art of medicine.

Sieglinde

What happened to the art of medicine?

Dr. Ongley

The art of medicine, particularly in the United States, has all but disappeared because machines have taken over. Have you had an x-ray, an MRI, a cat scan? Because the legal profession has made it so miserable for the medical profession that the doctor has to have record after record to back up the reason he made a particular decision.

I believe that in schooling young physicians, we should literally take them to the top of a mountain where there are no machines and bring the patients and say, "Please sit with these patients and figure out what is wrong with them" just to teach them the art of observation and examination without the aid of machines. I will talk to doctors today who have patients with back problems and I'll ask what's wrong with them and the first thing they say is "We will look at the x-ray."

There seems to be schooling in medicine—which drives me crazy—that if you look at a patient from the front we categorize, let's say, the head, the neck, a chest, a belly, pelvis, legs from the front. The patient complains of pain in the back. How often does the doctor walk around to the back of the patient to have a look? If he does go around to the back, does he then categorize the head, the back, et cetera? Then it's perfectly fine to take out all sorts of equipment—

knives, big needles—and stick them into someone's belly and do a parasynthesis or, if the person is pregnant, do an amniocentesis and stick a big needle right through the uterus down near where the baby is taking out fluid, or poking a catheter all the way up to the heart...and when you turn the patient around to the back, nothing. So we look at patients from the front relatively well but from the back very poorly. Energy moves through the body front and back yet the doctor will only look at the front.

The patient lying in a hospital bed with acute pain in his belly or chest, the doctor will localize the belly or chest area and determine the origin of that patient's pain. Now the same patient is lying in the same bed face up with a pain in his back...the doctor doesn't even turn him over. Why? I have no explanation for this, I am simply pointing out the errors. Teach people to look at patient from all sides, whichever is the best for the patient.

If we came upon an island which had not been previously discovered and the people who lived there did not have any knowledge of modern medicine and someone complained of a pain in the front, they would be just as confused as the person who complained of the pain in the back. They haven't made the progress of dividing it up into sections to find out which organ in what part of the body is complaining. Let's face it, it is very confusing from the front. There are many structures that could go wrong. Yet we have found a certain pathway through the jungle from the front. Turn them over and we have no pathways. Why not?

My criticism would let us evaluate the results of any particular species of physician very fairly. Evaluate fairly and let's get rid of this sort of medicine that I, as a physician, could not point my finger at my colleague. We would all know the results of specific treatments for specific ailments. These things are not published. What *is* published is how many people die from heart disease. Our treatment programs are not evaluated.

Sieglinde

This is part of a much bigger problem. The propagation and doom and gloom and negativity all around us. The victimization in our society.

Dr. Ongley

This is what sells. What I am trying to do here is change that thought. Let us look at things from a different point of view. As you well know I am happy to look at the blue sky and the beautiful white clouds and feel the tropical breeze on me. This is very pleasant. This is wonderful. This, however, is not making me ten million dollars on the stock market—so what is more important, making ten million dollars or appreciating life? The answer seems obvious. Why, then, do we have millions and millions of people who concentrate on the ten million dollars every day. Whether they ever get it or not is not the issue. Life is not appreciated. Our values are incorrect. All we need to do is get our feet firmly on the ground and learn what is the value of life.

I mentioned to you last night when you stand before Mr. and Mrs. God and they say, "What have you done with your life to make yourself happy?" You were rather confused by the question. When you analyze it, you have done very little. So if life is to be enjoyed, let's find out what makes life enjoyable and pursue it. That doesn't mean to be harmful to other people because what we do must be modulated. So what we should be looking at is what makes the majority truly happy.

Sieglinde

Having been in medicine for over sixty years, what has been your greatest happiness?

Dr. Ongley

Relieve people of discomfort, restore any physical abnormality to the normal so they are able to approach life without pain and without handicap.

Sieglinde

How have you learned this?

Dr. Ongley

Developing the philosophy of what life is all about. What is important in life? Remember there is tremendous power in truth and simplicity.

Sieglinde

Why have so few physicians figured out the simplicity of life?

Dr. Ongley

I don't have a crystal ball, but as of yet it has not been figured out. Exclude all of the worldly wealth. What would make you happy today? So that when you went to bed tonight you would say to yourself, "Yes, I feel bliss and had a great day."

. . .

I once told you a story of a Russian ex-circus strongman, an elderly man, who looked at least thirty years younger than his chronological age and he told me he was going off to a certain country to enjoy himself. I challenged him by saying, "This is the place for me to go, not for you to go." He said, "No, no, no, it's the place for me to go" and we went round and round with this for a long time and I finally asked him, "Please, what is the secret of life as you found it?"

The secret of life, as you have found it, is to enable you at your particular age to be thinking the way you think, acting the way you're acting, doing the things you're doing, and he finally confided in me and he said, "The secret of life, is doing what you want to do when you feel like doing it, providing it does not harm others."

Sieglinde

Isn't this truly the biggest question today? Everyone is looking to find himself, his path, his purpose, his reason for existing. How do we find this? What makes doing what you have passion for so difficult?

Dr. Ongley

Simply do as you want when you want when you feel like it, providing it hurts no one. This is very responsible and is this not our birthright to be happy.

Sieglinde

We do need to make money and take care of our family.

. . .

Dr. Ongley

Why have jobs you don't like and why make taking responsibility for the children you choose to bring into the world a burden? It is a choice that you make. When people don't do this, they have the idea that Mr. God and Mrs. God decreed that they should suffer.

These are the very people who feel more pain and hold more anxiety, fear, stress, and disease in the physical body. Take the story of my Russian strongman—when he gets up there and he's asked the question, "I gave you this blessing of life, you were to enjoy it. Did you?" He will say, "Heck yes." The big chief will say, "How did you manage that?" "I did what I wanted to do when I felt like doing it, provided I harmed no one."

At that particular point in time when I spoke with him, he was off to Bali, and when he returned he came in to see me. As soon as he came in the door, he posted his anger at me and burst out laughing; he pranced around the room like an absolute idiot and he still had his finger extended toward my nose and he said, "See, I did what I wanted to do when I wanted to do it and I really enjoyed myself. I didn't harm anyone. What did you do? Did you do what you felt like doing when you wanted to?"

And my answer was "Yes, I did." I had a lot of people who needed my help and I healed them all and I was disgustingly happy. He pulled down that pointing finger and said, "By gosh you learned it, something I had known for many, many years."

. . .

I am not original, what did William Shakespeare say—"He that giveth is twice blessed"?

Sieglinde

Most people live in a me-me-me society. How can you help them?

Dr. Ongley

Sit with them, discuss things, let them read about it, and when their time to wake up comes they will wake up to their own bliss. We are talking about normal rational human beings, not the insane —that would be a waste of time.

Sieglinde

Where did you grow up?

Dr. Ongley

In my parents' home in New Zealand. I was the baby. I had one sister and five brothers and we all became physicians.

Sieglinde

How far back can you remember?

Dr. Ongley

I remember being six months old and I remember being happy.

Sieglinde

How do you know it was happiness?

Dr. Ongley

I didn't know happiness was labeled, it just is, isn't it? I felt warmth and contentment. I remember trying to stand up and things like that. How far back can you remember?

Sieglinde

You are a very outstanding man with great gifts—what makes you so special?

Dr. Ongley

Wait a minute, you did not answer my question? How far back can you remember?

Sieglinde

Two to three. I do remember for an instant being born and lying on a blanket on the floor noticing no one was there and feeling upset and abandoned.

Dr. Ongley

Well, great. When we talk about memories let's not get confused thinking this is about what we had for breakfast yesterday. We have memories and I don't know if I have memories of my birth or if I heard stories of my birth and remember those. I remember coming from the dark to the light.

Sieglinde

I understand. My brief birth experience came when my mother's sister passed away and my mother and I made a trip to Germany to manage the home I was born in and empty its contents. Many childhood memories rushed through me during that month. I asked my mother to show me exactly where I was born after the midwife came. I laid a blanket on that spot in the upstairs room. Pictures of that moment came very clearly and I saw and felt them as if I was floating above the tiny wide-eyed baby. She was sad and upset, feeling alone and uncared for. She did not know her mother's bleeding could not be stopped and all tended to this crisis. I held this in my memory my entire life.

It is interesting that you say from the dark to the light. Most people believe it to be the other way around. You make it appear as if you came from elsewhere with a clear mission to perform.

Dr. Ongley
Yes I was.

Sieglinde
The light is the birth.

Dr. Ongley
Yes, sure it is.

Sieglinde
When you were a little boy, did you know you came to heal others?

. . .

Dr. Ongley

No one ever knows what they are supposed to do with their life —what do those words mean? I think all of us are here to heal; most of us ignore it and few will take the steps and be recognized as a healer as some people today call a doctor. As long as I can remember I have always wanted to help, whether it was an injured cat or dog, I did not like seeing a cat who looked to me to be suffering. Same applies to human beings. I want to help. I very definitely do not want to harm anyone. I see a smirk on your face. Did you ever in your formative years want to pull the wing out of a fly, or stick something into an injured cat, or harm anything?

Sieglinde

Of course not, never. I do have an experience after I started a school in the Bay Area. There was a little boy who pulled the tail out of a rabbit and left a bloody hole. He is in prison now.

Dr. Ongley

Then you are well aware that there are creatures on this earth who love inflicting pain. There are wolves who want to gobble up other injured wolves. How come you didn't want to do that?

Sieglinde

I don't have an answer, I just would never do that.

Dr. Ongley

Then wouldn't it be foolish to turn to someone who had a similar experience as you to ask them when did you know you were a healer?

. . .

I am saying that with your abilities and expertise, much of which you are denying, you know that such things are not a conscious decision. You are either that way from the beginning or you are not.

People who are not seem to assiduously practice their habitual ways, and too few of us spend a great deal of time perfecting their arts or attempting to perfect their arts in helping people, be it mental suffering or financial suffering, whatever it happens to be.

Sieglinde

On a planet of duality, doesn't it make sense that both exist and are a reflection of one another?

Dr. Ongley

This may be a reality but it doesn't make sense. Suppose we walk outside of this hotel and someone says to us, "Buddy, can you spare a dime?" What is your first reaction?

Sieglinde

I would give it to him. Then I would think, *Will this really help him or am I just enabling the habit of begging?*

Dr. Ongley

Does this classify you as a helper? If a hundred people were asked, "Buddy, can you spare a dime?" what would their first thought be? In the vernacular of today, we are born softies yet everyone really needs help.

. . .

Sieglinde

I am having a real problem with you. I sense you are without ego. You downplay your uniqueness; you share genius and gifts that you carry in your heart for the people of the world. You patiently sit while I ask you one thing after another.

Dr. Ongley

What do you consider ego, self-respect? This is what ego really is, and yes I have an ego because I have self-respect. I could not have self-respect if I intentionally harmed anyone.

Sieglinde

Your humility and simplicity overwhelm me and bring tears to my eyes.

Dr. Ongley

So what, must I be complicated? I am to be judged. I am not a judge myself. If what you say is true, these are your opinions; there may be others who disagree with you and you can have a discussion with them about it whether you are correct or he is.

Sieglinde

The truth about you remains the same no matter what anyone else thinks.

Dr. Ongley

In my opinion, yes.

. . .

Sieglinde

Have you always had a gift to heal and to see people for who they are?

Dr. Ongley

Seeing people for what they are is very different from healing. I have always had a desire to help. In this society, which is dominated by money, that isn't necessarily the best way to become affluent. I can never sit down and say that my life is dictated by having a massive fortune. Of course I would like to have that but would prefer to lead my life the way I lead it and let the money come.

Sieglinde

If you had a hundred million dollars, how would your life be different?

Dr. Ongley

I could help more people, I could educate more people with similar thoughts, who in turn could treat multitudes of people. Unfortunately to help people it takes money to facilitate helping more. Most physicians want to help. They just don't know how. Some become physicians for the prestige associated with the title, ego, power, control, money. Here is the ego. Yes, Mary wants to be a doctor. If people who came along are silly enough to listen to them, I supposed they feel powerful at the expense of the many powerless people.

You also can't have the other end of the spectrum and sit cross-legged on the mountain top in Nepal and talk about nothingness achieving Zen; this is absolute nothingness. Heck no. When Mr.

God and Mrs. God ask you, "What did you do with this gift called life?" Well, I sat cross-legged on the mountain top in Nepal. I don't think you've learned anything because you have achieved nothing even though you did what you wanted when you wanted and hurt no one. Nothing can be applied to nothing. If my mission is to contribute to life and help, then I better get off the mountain and roll up my sleeves and get on with it. The world must turn and everyone must play their part.

Sieglinde

How can the medical profession see more and care more?

Dr. Ongley

By patients being better acquainted with themselves so they expect more from the physician. As we mentioned previously, not to accept things that are obviously foolish. Treating a part of the body which is not abnormal. So we demand high standards of care from our physicians.

Sieglinde

How do the victims of the world fit into the scheme of things?

Dr. Ongley

Point out to them that the world does not owe them anything and that they have been given the same gift of life, and it is to be enjoyed. Considering themselves victims, they are not enjoying the gift. They have to get it through their heads and into their souls that they have the gift of life and it is to be enjoyed and not to be suffered. When they get up the big steps and are asked the question what did they do with their gift, now the whimpering and the reasons begin. Hey man, sorry you failed the test. You go down the stairs and rerun. Life is a test! A test of yourself.

Sieglinde

Too many people feel life is about accumulation, a relationship, that soul mate, and once I have that, I am whole and happy.

Dr. Ongley

When you mention relationship, why do people crave relationships? Isn't it a generational thing? Who started the story that you are supposed to get all the pebbles at your end of the beach? We perpetuate it. Now that you have accumulated all of the pebbles, can you even hold on to them. Does it make you happy or do you just want more and then the neighbor's pebbles? What's the point? Are you happy?

Sieglinde

What makes it so uncomfortable for people to know your greatness?

Dr. Ongley

Because I'm vulnerable like everyone else.

Sieglinde

I would think that you would gain happiness from your greatness.

Dr. Ongley

Pride is a form of sin, isn't it?

Sieglinde

You obviously have a mission, came here with remarkable gifts as did Pasteur, Einstein, and many great man who were sent here before the world was ready for them. Where are you from and who sent you?

Dr. Ongley

Do you know? If you asked Albert, he would tell you he was from Germany. Now if you are implying that there is a divine order, or someone delineates these things, then the answer would have to be yes.

Sieglinde

Other than being a doctor, are there other options for you?

Dr. Ongley

The only option I have is to die. I am who I am and I don't have a choice.

Sieglinde

If you had one dream that would come true today, what would it be?

Dr. Ongley

To be happy. Happy is a comparative. I could be happier by

helping more people. The world's most complexing problems yield to the onslaught of simplicity.

Sieglinde

Why is it so complex?

Dr. Ongley

It is complex because people are seeking the answers. If you have a multiplicity of people attacking one problem with different so-called solutions, you now have a complex mess of nothing and then when someone comes along with a very simple answer, the complexity vanishes.

Sieglinde

In your case, this might not be true. You have a simple answer and you are chastised for it.

Dr. Ongley

You see, the *inteligencia* maintain that simple answers are too simple initially and then they see the light, they accept it and that's it.

Sieglinde

Talk about medical school.

Dr. Ongley

Medical school is always very difficult. The quantity of so-called facts that one must assimilate. If you look at greater anatomy alone, there are over two hundred facts on each and every page and there are fifteen to seventeen hundred pages. That's a tremendous number of facts that should be known. Because it beholds anyone who is going to spend their time in trying to help the human body, we should say mind and body then you should know what the body is composed of. If you don't, as we mentioned yesterday, you come upon an island of people who have no perception of what we call modern medicine they haven't in our measure made very much progress in the treatment of human ailments. We may come upon another island where they are so much more advanced than we are. A simple case, a very simple place.

Sieglinde

If devouring such masses of information, why are you still sixty-plus years later reading and studying medicine each day?

Dr. Ongley

Well, it is important to stay up to date about how the other person thinks. Someone once said, "If you meet a man and you don't understand his language and he does not understand your language, then to you he is ignorant and you to him are ignorant." You have got to have a common basis of communication.

Sieglinde

So what you're saying, then, is that for you to teach others and invite them in helping people, you must speak to ears that can listen and see from their eyes?

Dr. Ongley

Yes, it's a way of putting it. So they can see what I consider clearly the best way for the patient. Maybe I'm not correct. Well, let's face it, my views have changed over the last ten years. If you were sitting here talking to me ten years ago I might say A plus B equals D. Today, A plus B equals D plus E. We change as we are able to comprehend more.

Sieglinde

Is it true that each cell in the body replaces itself every seven years including the memory?

Dr. Ongley

When a cell changes, does it actually lose the ability to record memory? The answer is no.

Sieglinde

Hopefully in seven years we have learned something and our consciousness has grown so with new habits we are able to make better choices that are imprinted in the cells.

Dr. Ongley

Sure, we have learned something, but we are talking about memory? In seven years' time you won't be able to remember a conversation. As a human adapts to the changing environment, we must change our thinking to deal with, let's call it the new human. I'm not speaking in evolutionary periods of time but you mentioned yesterday that if you were suddenly thrust into the middle of India not comprehending the language and you were forced, I'm not saying with a sword at your back, it was necessary for you to earn a living working there, things would be very difficult. So we are asking young physicians to be suddenly thrust in the middle of India and deal with totally different ways they should be handling their patient.

Sieglinde

I hear you using the sword often. What are you really referring to?

Dr. Ongley

Wasn't there some Greek who solved the Gordian knot by cutting right through it. For years and years people tried to unravel it. Ulysses said no, and he pulled out the sword, and cut right through it. That was the end of the Gordian knot. This is not a literal sword but a metaphorical sword. I mean, if you are going to spend your entire lifetime on the outside of the problem, how on earth would you ever reach the core so you could understand and change it?

I'll give you an example of the arthroscopic approach to a joint. If you take the scope and push it into the joint, it's gone past many tissues and you are merely looking at the inside of the joint. Now we are here in what we might call a room and we push the arthroscope through the wall. There we would observe the inside of this room but supposing that the damage were in the roof or the walls, the scope has gone in beyond and you can't observe it. Yet today physicians say, "Oh you have a perplexing knee problem; I think we will we will have to go in with a scope and have a look," and the patient is actually thinking that the physician is actually looking at the entire knee. All he is doing is looking at the inside of the knee. Now you can fall down and get a marked abrasion but there is nothing wrong with the knee. There are many causes of pain in the knee itself. Yet we look at the arthroscope as the answer to a diagnosis. No it is not. It is a help.

Sieglinde

Then what is the answer to a correct diagnosis?

Dr. Ongley

It is the same as the diagnosis for any part of the body. You test its function. The function of the various structures. Now I'm not saying that the physician is so blind that he can't see a large abrasion on the skin involving maybe the subterranean tissues but supposing the damage was just beneath the skin, how is he going to solve that problem? He can't see it, he can't use his scope. It does not show up on an x-ray. Now he says, "Well okay, we'll do a cat scan or an MRI." These of course are stationary pictures and generally speaking it is when a tissue is stretched or twisted or something that cries out in pain. You are not getting a picture of what is causing the pain in that particular knee. You may get an image of the various structures but you are not in a position to identify what is making him cry out in pain.

If a physician may think there is something wrong with your heart, generally speaking he tests the function of the heart by having you walk to see if it beats a little faster or stops or what have you. He does a cardiac function test. If he suspects your liver, he will do the liver function tests. If he suspects the kidneys, he will do the kidney function tests and so on.

But when it comes to the back or the knee, he will take an x-ray of it and if it shows nothing he is confused and will go to the other types of scans which may be more detailed but not necessarily give him any diagnosis.

We all know that if you tighten the quadriceps the knee goes up and straight, and if you tighten the hamstrings the knee bends. You should be able to figure out is the pain coming from the attachment of the hamstring muscles or the attachment at the quadriceps muscles or what have you. We know that the various ligaments in the knee and in the walls of the knee as we will call it have a certain function. Ligament A will cause the knee to go this direction and ligament B will cause it to go the opposite direction so if you push it this way you would be testing that latency of these particular ligaments and slowly but surely by receiving negative, negative, negative responses—ah positive, negative, don't stop when you find a positive, negative, negative, positive. Now we find, of the more than one hundred structures in the knee, two malfunctioning and all the others are fine. So it would make sense to assume that the patient had damaged that one particular structure.

Sieglinde

In medical school, isn't a doctor learning all of this?

Dr. Ongley

No. In actual fact, he is not. To do the functional test the muscular skeleton system is time-consuming; it is boring and it doesn't truly fit the image of a supreme doctor. So he usually, if he suspects a thing like that, will do tests along the lines of an EMG or electromyographic testing or he will send the patient to a physical therapist to do muscle testing. The books on that particular subject do not point out that a muscle is weakest when it is on full stretch so most of the tests are done in the normal mutual position of the joint. Therefore you are not testing the full function of that particular structure unless initially you put it on a stretch.

Sieglinde

How did you discover this?

Dr. Ongley

When a muscle contracts, it contracts in little segments and when this one uses up all of its glycogen and can't contract anymore. The little segments of that muscle contracts, so obviously to get the full function of that muscle, you must not use it in the mid position. You are more likely to elicit pain if you put that biceps muscle on a full stretch and then ask it to contract against resistance.

So for the physiological principal of how a muscle functions, you are now able to say, "Let's test the muscle the correct way." If it's weak on its fully stretched position and you are suspecting something is malfunctioning in that muscle, put it into its weakest position and test it. If you put it into its strongest position, the tester will be deluded that the muscle is okay unless there is a huge gross problem with it, for example, if the biceps muscle is torn away.

Sieglinde

So because it is boring and time-consuming, they don't test the function.

Dr. Ongley

In their opinion they are doing more important things because the conditions of the muscular skeleton system don't kill people. Okay, so they are dealing with the more serious side of medicine, and I often say to people if they say to me they have a bad back, we have a wonderful play that can be observed and played out.

In the wonderful days of the Wild West when people pushed their wagons across the United States, don't you think there were people who injured their back or tore ligaments? Of course there were. What was the natural history of them—did they all die? If you push a wagon you might die of a heart attack or receive an arrow in the back. What happened to these fellows?

So you go to Tombstone, Arizona and you look at Boothill Cemetery and you look for a plaque that will read along the lines of, *Here lies Paul Mac, he didn't die from a .44 but bit the dust due to a pain in the back.* There is no such Tombstone there.

So the crappies did not die that way. So physicians are dealing with the crisis of life and death. I'm not dealing with that crisis. I'm dealing with a simple mundane thing called pain, which by the way, most all people have in their skeletal system.

Sieglinde
Pain, then, is not a serious enough problem in the medical system.

Dr. Ongley
To me, it is very serious, and to the patient it is very serious but to the doctor it is not. There are pills for pain. If he has a choice of

saving that man's life or taking care of that patient with the pain, the answer is quite obvious, isn't it?

Orthopedic doctors who have a patient who has suffered serious damage in a car accident, they must be dealt with quickly or the patient will go into shock and die. Their time if you must make a choice; life is a problem of economics. Now they have made the right choice.

However, my side of the discussion is that there should be a section of orthopedics who deal with those life and death situations. Also a section who deal simply with pain. Today there are pain clinics everywhere and fail when the pain is from the musculoskeletal system and the doctors prescribing pain pills to temporarily relieve symptoms but the cause was never treated or diagnosed so you end up with patients who become drug addicts in pain. There are many thousands and thousands of these people. If you have the opportunity to go to a pain clinic and see the daily volume of people seeing the poor doctor and he is at his wits end, what can he do? It's not really his fault.

Sieglinde
Whose fault is it?

Dr. Ongley
It is the fault that there are too few physicians in that particular field. This is why state medicine in principle is wonderful because there should be a physician for every ten or hundred people or whatever it happens to be. There should be adequate physicians to take care of all people. This is the object behind it.

. . .

Unfortunately, the human failing of greed comes in and the doctor says, "Why should I work like a slave over here while that chap there works on Wall Street from 9:00 to 4:00 making his millions and retires at an early age and has two Bentleys? I as a physician have not only the highest divorce rate in the world but lose ten years of my life simply by being in the profession that I'm in." He has given up half of his life going to medical school depending what country you are in. In the British countries eight years, then four years of medical school. Then you're back in residency for three years. Suddenly we are talking about eleven or twelve years and in all of that time the poor physician or his father is paying out or he has borrowed the money from the bank and then when does he go out there, there are not enough hospital positions so he goes into private practice. What does he have to do? He has to get a building, build an office, have nice cars and is eleven years behind in the money game, grossly in debt, and now if you are a young person you better have a wife. So now the guy has to have a wife. The wife of course wants a house, so now he has an office down here, and a house up on the hill. He's got no money, into the high rate of divorce, a shorter life span and if he doesn't do these things the patient or the medical profession says, "Oh he is no good." It is a vicious cycle.

Sieglinde

It seems that the only way he can make it is to see masses of people and charge a hefty fee.

Dr. Ongley

In the socialized scheme, the government will pay X number of dollars for every patient you see. Initially, you start out by being allowed to see an unlimited number of patients. He might see 100 or 150 each day, all at X number of dollars per patient. Now the government turns around and says he is making too much money and decrees that he can only see twenty-five to fifty people each day still at X number of dollars per patient. The competent doctor goes in every day, crashes through his patient load; it is now 2:00 in the afternoon; taxation is so high there is no point in continuing work or he has broken the law by seeing more than his quota so the good physician is out in the sunshine walking up and down not knowing what to do with himself. Obviously if you are going to be in what I call a sorting station, you don't have time. If you're going to see fifty patients a day, you don't have time to look after the seriously ill patients. You now become very good at sorting them out: "You stay; you go to the hospital. I'll stay here and look after the ingrown toenail," and he becomes very good at doing the minor procedures and sorting people out. When you have all the doctors in town doing that and there is one hospital, very soon of course the hospitals are filled with these referred patients and now you've got the doctors in the hospital overworked and not enough hospital beds. Please tell me the answer.

Sieglinde

We better wake up and take care of our own body and take responsibility for our optimal state of health.

Dr. Ongley

This is the most important thing. If you look at the United States, they have tried to regulate vitamins and health foods. Big Pharma regulates the information available that is of the highest benefit for us and makes the most money for them. The side of the discussion should be that the doctors' record was an expert. If you judge the physician on his results, he obviously is not an expert.

And as you mentioned, who knows your body better than yourself? So you should look after it as best you can, and after that, consult someone who knows more about it than you. You must, however, be awake and aware and ask the right questions and demand to know the cause of the problem and not settle for a bandage called a prescription.

It is wonderful that people are waking up and getting into health—let's get everyone into it. People would make healthier and wiser choices in all areas of their lives. If everyone was into health you wouldn't have the huge volume of obese and sick people. Now the number of physicians that we have would be able to cope with the problem. You still have the people who injure themselves, and for that you come to the musculoskeletal system and if it does not require dramatic medical interference, where does the patient go to get specific adequate therapy for the musculoskeletal system?

Look at the number of people in that field. You have the MDs, the chiropractors, the physical therapists, the osteopaths, muscular therapists, and many others.

Why is it that we have so many different health professionals in the same field? If they were curing them all, there wouldn't be enough patients to go around.

Sieglinde
    It sounds to me that there is much confusion in this field and professionals are attempting to fill their niche.

· · ·

Dr. Ongley

But we decided that there is a simple answer to every complicated problem. Are we making it more complicated by saying, "Oh this patient over here needs chiropractic care," whatever that is, which means manipulation. Now you have an argument. All of the modalities have manipulation of some kind. Or are they really all the same? If they are, let us get rid of the Gordian knot of manipulation and let's say all of these people are doing the same thing. And then all you have to do is teach the physician who is in medical school to manipulate. The indications for manipulation would eliminate the variety of people in this field.

Sieglinde

The professionals in this field also have a financial, as well as an ego survival mechanism to protect.

Dr. Ongley

Correct. Again, you must judge people by their results.

Sieglinde

Who would we appoint to do that daily? God?

Dr. Ongley

Mr. and Mrs. God would be very good but they don't come down here often enough to do this.

Sieglinde

I don't see this happening in any system. Honestly and fairly that is, with proper and fair consequences.

. . .

Dr. Ongley

I agree it will not happen, but is there any other test than results? If there is no other test then this must be used and we are back to basics and simple principles. Instead of chiropractors fighting with their peers, why don't they do a clinical study on the results?

Sieglinde

Why not have clinical studies that are unbiased showing the large percentage of people who die every year from the over-prescribed patient on prescription drugs? In the elderly I saw a study stating over eight percent of deaths are caused here.

Dr. Ongley

I agree. And this has been done. Goodman from Massachusetts wrote a very good book on the shoulder

and one of the things he insisted upon being a surgeon was that he would tabulate his own results. So he would know his results. He was rather alarmed at how poor his own results were, particularly when the other doctors in the hospital were bragging about their great results. So he insisted in the hospital that everyone's results were evaluated so they had a common language and knew what they were talking about.

Sieglinde

What happened to Dr. Goodman?

Dr. Ongley

They threw him out of the hospital. Then they threw him out of the medical society for proposing such an insane idea. Basically they all knew they were lying to themselves. Evaluate the performance of any hospital and you would be afraid to even walk into one. MDs believe that the institution is the greatest thing there is. This record is clear that one in every four patients receives the incorrect medication. This is a terribly high percentage. The sensible awake people will of course take a friend into the hospital with them and check everything that is being given to them by the nurse or the doctor himself.

Sieglinde
It sounds to me that no one cares.

Dr. Ongley
There is a lot of truth in that. It is easy to cover up in a hospital. If you were in private practice you were crucified. This is why I'm saying the *results* of *all* procedures should be public knowledge.

Sieglinde
Will this ever happen?

Dr. Ongley
If they evaluate you in your ability to drive a car, then why would it not be possible? It is much more likely if the masses of people insist on it.

Sieglinde
It seems people are asleep in their own lives.

. . .

Dr. Ongley

People have the power to change this, but most are too lazy. You have a vote and the day people in Washington, DC are made responsible for their action, you will get somewhere. When people take a stand along with the president and the first lady, then we have the power and become responsible for our actions and choices.

Sieglinde

Will people ever stand up in mass and say, "I have had it with all of this nonsense, I am not a sheep or a mushroom kept in the dark and fed bullshit—enough is enough"?

Dr. Ongley

Of course there are many incidents in history where people did stand up. Let's talk about the Boston Tea Party or let's get a little more serious the French Revolution. The people stood up, but the problem is the next group to go into power are still human and just as corrupt. This is why I do not consider myself fit to rub shoulders with the human race. This is one of the reason for corruption. You used the term yesterday me-me-me and that's all people are interested in. No one cares about progress. Go back to Shakespeare and man's inhumanity to man.

Sieglinde

Are you implying that man is basically corrupt?

Dr. Ongley

Yes.

Sieglinde

Is this how man is supposed to be?

Dr. Ongley

I'm not God. I was simply sent to help and heal. I really don't believe it is supposed to be that way, but it is, isn't it?

We have a book of rules called the Bible just as we have a book of rules for people who drive cars. If everyone

followed the rules, things would be pretty good but people in general don't because again of the me-me-me.

Sieglinde

We have policemen and laws.

Dr. Ongley

What kind of person falls in the category of policeman? Why does he fall into this category? Does he want to carry a gun? In the United States, if someone doesn't do as I tell them, I shoot them. Is this the type who becomes a policeman? Unfortunately yes, so we know he has the potential for being corruptible.

Sieglinde

Getting back to physicians, what *don't* they learn in medical school?

. . .

Dr. Ongley

Again, we are back to the problem of economics. There is only a certain amount of time you can force people to go to medical school so you must choose the gravity of the knowledge and the situation that must be taught to train those people, otherwise you would be in medical school for twenty-five years.

Sieglinde

Yesterday you spoke at length about observing people. What would be so difficult and time-consuming

about teaching that? It seems to me this is a very basic principle and truth in all situations.

Dr. Ongley

In my day in medical school you were asked by your teacher to go into the hospital ward and just look around and go outside and tell the teacher which one was a cardiac patient, a liver patient, a kidney patient just by looking at their faces. This is a well-recognized art in medicine. Today, however, in medicine you cannot practice the art. You must practice a so-called science. We discuss medicine.

Sieglinde

A plastic surgeon considers himself an artist.

Dr. Ongley

I don't know what he considers himself to be. He is trying to alter, to shape, and form on the human body. Of course, he has to face the age-old problem that her big toe is not the shape she thinks it should be and she is dictating, "I am employing you to do it."

Sieglinde

Isn't it a shame that more people are not dictating what is proper inside their body in everyday life, setting cosmetics aside? This is a whole other issue.

Dr. Ongley

There is goodness in all people if given the correct opportunity. Unfortunately, the way our civilization has evolved, many good people are not given the opportunity to express this goodness. I had a call from friends in Tennessee the other night and the conversation was along these lines. It seems that the only way to get along today in the United States is to be a crook. Being straightforward and honest doesn't seem to bring the big results most people want.

Sieglinde

I disagree. Success and great success is possible with complete honestly and integrity. You must, however, be willing to pay the price and to understand that you may not fit in and expect an uphill fight. But at least you are playing your game and living your life with purpose, being an example for others. Why else are those who are helpers here?

Dr. Ongley

Again, I said it *seems* to be, not necessarily always is. I said to my friend in Tennessee, "But you can't be that way" and he said, "No I can't. Everything I do is controlled by the bureaucracy and it is corrupt. Therefore you bribe them if you want to achieve a result, or you don't." This is why he said "seems."

Sieglinde

If you are committed you either find a way or you do something else.

Dr. Ongley

Not necessarily. If you are in construction or a coal mine, someone has to do it. The set of rules has to be followed by the book of rules whether you like it or not. Otherwise you have a freeway falling down or a coal mine collapsing.

Sieglinde

How did you develop your set of rules and the Ongley technique? It is in all of the medical journals and you have been treating patients all over the world. Last week you were invited to teach a group of medical professionals in Italy. What is the medical technique?

Dr. Ongley

There is not one single entity as the Ongley technique. There are many, many different techniques that I have had to develop. You have the patient there and the patient doesn't respond now you must do something else. If you are referring to the Ongley technique for reduction of sacroiliac joint with dislocation and treating bad backs then there is a very simple answer, and I do of course remember the first person I used it on. It was in New Zealand and a friend of mine was playing rugby football. He was tackled by many people from different angles on the field and he damaged his back and was carried to me on a stretcher. I played and coached rugby so I was the obvious choice.

I looked at him and had him x-rayed and did all of the classical things. We talked yesterday of people with bad backs who are lying on their backs when they are being examined, as it was with this poor chap. He was lying on his back in very acute pain. He was remarkably deviated—his hip stuck out to one side, so after a lot of time he tried to stand and with great difficulty he did and was markedly deviated. The classical test of straight leg raises to indicate if there was pressure on the nerve. He was very positive I could barely lift his leg off the couch; he screamed in severe pain in the lower back area and down his right leg.

The x-ray was negative but the classical test of weakness of hamstring muscles, the gastrocnemius muscles, the diminished ankle jerk, and diminished sensation in the S1 distribution down his leg were all present. I said, "Brian, your rugby days are over." He looked at me in horror. "What do I do?" "You can lie in bed for six weeks and see if the pressure on the nerve goes away or you can have traction or surgery." Again, in any case he would never play again.

He said, "Why don't you do to my back what you did to my shoulder last week?" The week before he had a dislocation in his shoulder. I did not like giving people general anesthesia but through the suggestion of this patient to use it on the part of the back that was causing him I did. I turned him on his tummy and spent forty-five minutes with a very long needle and a large bottle of local anesthetic and very slowly infiltrated the various tissues from the skin on, and after forty-five minutes and putting in a rather large volume of anesthetic, I noticed that he was simply lying on his stomach talking to me and turning his head as if he had no pain at all. Then I said, "Well Brian I put it in, and you have no pain." I can't even stop him—he took no notice of me! He got up on his own two feet and started to bend down and touch his toes, which he was able to do full range with no pain after two or three attempts. "I'm fine," he said. I laid him down on the couch. I re-did all of the tests. Testing the strength of his muscles—all tests were now normal. Even the decreased sensation in the skin was normal. I didn't know back then whether this was temporary or whether he was actually back to normal. From the academic understanding of it, none of it made any sense.

All doctors are well aware that if one does a straight leg test and the patient is markedly limited then the most frequent cause is pressure on the nerve root. The most common cause for pressure on the nerve root is displacement or partial displacement of the disc. So either I put the disc back into place so I stretched the nerve— which is very unlikely, because it was still functioning. Either I had taken the disc and put it back in place or somehow had gotten the disc back into and put it back in place or somehow had gotten the disc away from the nerve. That was how I was analyzing it and of course I couldn't possibly do anything to the sacroiliac articulation because they are categorically stated in medicine. They do not move they are set down together by ligaments. It is impossible to move them. They will break in half before they move. They never subluxate, they never ever dislocate unless there is an accompanying fracture, but there is no accompanying fracture. This is what I was taught in medicine. It turned out to be incorrect.

The most common cause of pain in the back is a malfunction of the sacroiliac articulation. I had learned many years ago when I was going to be a specialist in obstetrics and gynecology and in all seriousness I was looking at a patient with my chief in the hospital in Dublin, Ireland. The patient was in agony with pain in her back. She was eight months pregnant.

In all seriousness I said, "What is actually causing her back pain?" The chief took me outside in horror and said, "You must be crazy, she is pregnant." But I've seen a lot of other pregnant patients and they all don't have pain in their back. It's not a normal accompaniment of pregnancy. Of course he being the chief and I being the humble student turned away from me and walked away and left me standing there.

I saw the same patient after she had come to term and had her baby. She was attending the outpatient clinic and she was still complaining of very severe back pain. Again I said to the chief, "Look, remember the patient, she's had the baby but still has the back pain." Again the chief took me outside reprimanded me and said, "Look, she has had the baby; this is why she has back pain."

So I gave up and I did not investigate the mechanism of pain. No one cared for this poor woman. They said the pregnancy did it, now live with it. Of course today we know that the pelvis is so narrow that generally speaking the head of the fetus will not go through the pelvic outlet without the hormone called relaxin, which causes the ligaments to be able to stretch so that when the head is coming down through the canal and coming to the outlet and rotating, these ligaments are able to stretch and allow bones to move apart so the head can go through, but unfortunately because we used to leave patients in the nursing mothers position there was no support from the muscles of the ligaments. The characteristic ligament that, when exposed, continue to stretch.

So if the ligaments that hold your knees together create an unstable knee...if the ligaments that hold your pelvis together, you have an unstable pelvis. When you put it on a mechanical disadvantage, it moves.

Sieglinde
So this is true of any joint.

Dr. Ongley
Yes and what I do is restore the normal function of the joint and then strengthening whatever tissues are stretched, causing the instability. It is very interesting to note that way back in 1934 in the *New England Journal of Medicine* there appeared an article by a Dr. Rice where he had investigated the injection result. His were the injection results for hernias.

So he got a lot of patients and much to his surprise he found we have occipitated a lot of scar tissue. Scar tissue is unyielding and held the hernia in place, which is what we needed. To his surprise we also found that we proliferated new tissue and where the tissue is attached to bone the area of attachment has become larger.

I said, "You know, chap, for the first time we are able to cause regeneration of tissues in the human body, which we thought we could not regenerate."

. . .

And so his book was read by Louie Shelts up in Canton, Ohio and Louie was an oral surgeon and an M.D. who was struck with this problem of the temperventicular joints so he began to inject a proliferating solution into the joints... And to his horror, in a series of nineteen [patients]—which he published—they all got well. He thought about this for twenty years and in his investigations. Not only did this synovial joint get well when he biopsied it, most of the tissues had become normal. synovial membrane had become normal, the disc inside the joint was normal, and the ligaments around the joints were normal. So all of this grinding down of teeth and pulling them out and all of the work that dentists have done since 1936 in spite of the fact.

Loui had published his findings. So other people in the world say, "Wow," and you always get someone who wants to ride on someone's back in the same town was George Hackett in Canton who was a surgeon. He published his work in 1956 a monograph on prophetic therapy, but of course like too many of these doctors, he said, "I've got twenty years of experience and this is no nonsense."

This happens too often in medicine. I knew George, he was a good guy, and very interested in the work he was doing. I did not understand the principles of testing the functions of the musculoskeletal system. He would go around and prod you and if it hurt he would stab you with his solution. And unfortunately the solution that he used was known as sylnenol, which was ilium seed oil, which caused such severe pain, and in George's own words, when you get a patient, you better treat everywhere because you will never get another shot at it. Then he would throw him in the hospital, put him under morphine, and if the guy woke up, the pain is gone and goodbye, that is it.

. . .

This painful procedure so handicapped progress in this field. Then you had others who would emulate what George was saying and inject necks with peculiar solutions and on record they killed two and caused temporary paralysis in three others, which of course caused medical professions to judge others by these procedures and not their own. They however cheerfully performed procedures that caused death left and right but that's okay. So what they imply and say is that the unestablished procedure must be wrong.

It wasn't until my solution came along—which didn't cause pain, and didn't have side effects—that it could be used in volume. We were able to make real progress in this field. There were many torrid times after lengthy experimentation when I first used it on human volunteers. You lie someone down on their tummy and put this into their lower back area. How did you know it wouldn't act like a hydrochloric acid and burn a hole all the way through? So when the patient said, "Oh I feel this is. I never went to sleep," I went rushing off to see how the patient was. So today it is very different for people getting into this field. I have done it with impunity and they don't have to go through the horror that we originators went through.

Sieglinde

So people come in have a treatment, walk out, and feel fine.

Dr. Ongley

Look at poor George Hackett. He was giving you morphine and shuffling you to the hospital or he did it in the hospital.

Sieglinde

I would think these patients were still not well, more likely worse off than before.

Dr. Ongley

This is correct. I used to laugh at George and tell him he belongs to the finger prodders association. He would prod you and if it hurt, he would stab you. Then he would say to me, "Ongley, laying on of hands, the laying on of hands." I would say, "George, you know it is so good stabilizing the joint if it's out of position." George of course didn't know how to evaluate a joint to see if it was out of position. So I say, "I have to lay on hands?"

The very last time I saw George Hackett before he died was in Atlantic City. We went out on the boardwalk together and laughed and joked like two good friends would do. He was very tall and I am very small. He was screaming at me even then, "Oh Ongley, the laying on of hands!" and I said, "George from the finger prodders association. We've got to get together and make progress in this field. This is how progress in this field in the United States came about!"

In 1959 or 1960 the prolotherapy association was formed and the first meeting was held in Washington, DC and I came from New Zealand to attend. I gave to George Hackett the solution known as Ongley solution. George went crazy on me. Ongley said, "George, you are up there giving the big speech with all of these other people here backing you up? You only have one chance with the patient; you better do everything. Here is a solution that basically does not hurt," and he was arguing with me thinking it was no good.

. . .

The way proliferin works, it initiates an inflammatory response within the body, and an inflammatory response is supposed to be painful so therefore it can't possibly work. I said, "Wait George, there is an ingredient in here named phenol, and it has a selective activity on mixed nerves which knocks out the pain-sensing fibers, leaving the motor fibers so the person can walk or do whatever they have to do and not feel the pain."

At the same time there was a man named Peterson, a physician who was doing a series of studies under George Hackett's watchful eye on the effect of the injection of proliferin on various soft tissues. To the best of my knowledge the only published study that halfway through the study they switched solutions and that was published in 1962 called injection therapy. So half was used the old solutions and the other half was the Ongley solutions in the middle. There was something very dramatic that occurred. George took the bottle and he tested it and said, "Oh my God, this really works."

Sieglinde

I am surprised everyone is not using it.

Dr. Ongley

How do you do it? You can't spread knowledge. You cannot stand up in a medical meeting and say, "Look, you chaps are all wrong. You're doing surgery on discs and discs don't occur in the frequency that you think they occur." Way back when in 1937 Mixter and Barr wrote a paper in which they identified and described discs pursing on the spinal cord and the nerve root as the causation of back pain and sciatica down the leg. So everyone jumps on the discogenic theory of the origin of back pain and pain down the limb.

. . .

However, again in 1936, Sir Thomas Lewis was fooling around looking at patients from the front and he kept getting pain so he thought he would inject an irritant into the soft tissue around the spine and into the pelvis. To his surprise he got a dull ache at the site of the injection which clearly defined repeatable pain spreading down the limb. So he said, "My God, pain is felt elsewhere other than at its source," which is truly referred pain as opposed to transferred pain down a nerve. Here he was injecting soft tissues producing pain similar to the pain of transferred pain down nerves but he was not injecting nerves, so he was proving that pain is spread widely in the human body in distances other than down a nerve. This is of paramount importance in explaining why the amputee can have a heart attack and have the pain down a limb which isn't even there.

It was very interesting, for instance, that they took a shoulder blade and took a bit of bone that sticks up the spine with the scapula and they injected it near the area of pain and he moved it just a wee bit from the spine just an inch away and got no pain in the shoulder blade but a pain elsewhere. Then you put the anesthetic in the area and the pain goes away.

Sieglinde

We mentioned people taking responsibility for their bodies and you see a patient with a pain in the knee, for example. What is the body communicating to the person? We know all organs and system have a language for the person. Example, the liver holds the emotion of anger and rage.

. . .

Dr. Ongley

Before we get around to that let us look at patient education and not letting a doctor treat the wrong area. Every ladies magazine that you pick up and every newspaper that you pick up there is something about discogenic theory and the pain in your neck going down your arm. Or the pain in your back going down your leg. If you ask your physician, "Give me another alternative diagnosis other than the disc," he simply cannot. It does not exist. But why is it since 1936 we have had all of the experimental work done first in Great Britain with Calvin's work with Sir Thomas Lewis, and Steifer in the United States? It's all there. If you have a pain that is spreading down the limb, it is not necessarily due to a disc. How come when this is all there it is not accepted?

Sieglinde

It's all about money and there is no money in all people being healthy.

Dr. Ongley

Yes. You have read the story about the French Revolution. All about *The Scarlet Pimpernel*, they see him here and they see him there. The is how I liken the discogenic theory—it has become the Scarlet Pimpernel. They see it here, they see it there, they see the damned disc everywhere and even when they can't identify it the doctor shouts out, "I can't find you but I know you're in there somewhere. I will go and look for it!" Why, why, why. Why doesn't he say, "Sir Thomas Lewis did such and such"? And there is the pain and I will take out my bottle of anesthetic and I will put it into the tissue as Thomas Lewis indicated. I put it in and as the pain goes. I don't have a disc and I don't have to operate on this poor person. This to me is inexcusable at this time. If you can educate people through writing or whatever that they need to say to the doctor,

"Just because I have a pain, it does not mean that my disc is disintegrating. My pain just came on. How could my disc have been disintegrating for years? What happened?"

Doctors, are you aware that there are other mechanisms of pain in the back and down the limb? Let's check those out and don't just keep checking the same disc. The doctor might say, "But all of the machines show this." But Doctor, you haven't even looked at the mechanism as the causation for the pain like the one I have.

When this hits the media, people will wake up very quickly because millions and millions of people are suffering with the problems I am referring to. Look at President Kennedy. One diskette for me, two diskettes for me, spinal graph, wear a corset, sit in a rocking chair. Such a failure of American medicine is a bloody joke. All of the information was there.

In other words, if we evaluate our results daily... Let's say I'm correct, then evaluate my results. Give me 100 patients and give the other physician 100 patients with his technique, and let's evaluate the results and accept them. If he is not the winner it needs to be looked at more carefully and reckoned with but he won't do that. Why must we always be lording a particular method just because someone was trained in it? And it makes a lot of money when it is not helping the patient.

We can look at the general make-up and characteristic of the average physician and you have had enough experience to know that if a doctor can get a better result he will do whatever it takes to get a better result. They are doing what they believe helps the patient the most. It may be incorrect. Their motivation is not to harm the patient, but to help the patient. However, it is difficult sometimes to change habits and sometimes there is not the time to learn and perfect a new technique.

Sieglinde

Why so much pain in the first place? Millions and millions of people. How does this happen?

Dr. Ongley

The causation of the pain is that the little nerves are stimulated. Either damaged, stretched, or twisted by something or from the release of certain chemicals in the body that trigger the mechanism. Then the pain goes up the nerve into the spinal cord where we have certain modulating influences that can make it worse and it is transferred to parts of the brain. We mentioned the memory and the conceptual, emotional, and visceral hormonal responses that accompany it. In the brain itself there are modulating influences just as there are in in the spinal cord, so what you feel is not really an indicator of the extent or the degree of the damage. What you feel is merely the result of how much modulation has been on that impulse getting up to the brain and the effects of the emotion on it.

Any experienced physician will tell you that the degree of pain that the patient is suffering has nothing or very little to do with the degree of damage in the body. You have two people with identical damage in the body and one suffers terribly and one a little. This is how we feel pain. It is either an indicator that the nerve endings have been triggered by compression, squeezing, twisting, or damage, or the release of chemicals from damaged tissues which trigger the little nerve endings and finally in the cortex area of the brain.

What you were asking previously in a very guarded way was, "Is the pain a defense mechanism?" You put your finger in the fire and pulled it out. Pain is an unpleasant emotional experience. The lesson to be learned is the patient's emotional state, either due to present or past experience, has a tremendous influence on what he or she is feeling.

Sieglinde

Where is the soul in the body? Or is it?

Dr. Ongley

There is. I have no concrete scientific proof. What color is the soul? There was a Russian experiment many years ago where they concluded that whatever life was on a scale upon death, he weighed less and it was assumed it was the soul [that departed]. I haven't seen one—have you?

Sieglinde

Do you have to see it to believe it? I have years of hospice experience and have seen and experienced the process of death hundreds of times as it happens and the process is consistently the same. I have felt the frequency of the soul. I felt a thickness, a change in the air around me. It was soft but thicker than before it appeared from the body. It is wispy at the same time and gives off a feeling of comfort or a calling to follow somehow. There are no words in our language to describe the feeling of it.

. . .

I have had the same feeling when holding grandchildren seconds after birth while holding them. It pours from their eyes as if they saw everything inside and outside of me.

Dr. Ongley

I would love to see it. Can you smell it?

Sieglinde

I have had no experience of a smell. I have seen one patient seconds before death sit up straight in bed hissing, and the wall behind his bed including his body turned a dark orange color. The nurse and I who were in the room froze like a statue as we watched the patient slide back into a laying position and take his last breath. I did not stay and went home. The energy in the room was painful and tearing into my energy field.

Dr. Ongley

For me, things need to be tangible to be real. Many have tried to program me about the soul but I need tangible evidence.

Sieglinde

I doubt that you will until you experience leaving your body. Your soul along with your life experiences and personality throughout all incarnations remains with you.

What is a human body other than energy?

Dr. Ongley

Is there more matter or more space?

Sieglinde

Space. With eyes who see, it is all energy and the matter an illusion. So the answer is more space from my point of view and experience with others. How does a tulip bulb know to be a tulip? When to grow and when to return to the soil? It is programmed with a frequency that is called "tulip ness." The same is true for a lemon, orange, or grapefruit tree. The lemon tree will not have grapefruit hanging from its branches. A human will not grow up to be a cat. The frequency from where we come is an energetic program guiding who and what we are.

Dr. Ongley

More space is correct.

Sieglinde

Yes, and since energy can't be destroyed, what happens to it at death?

Dr. Ongley

Sir Isaac Newton says energy can't be destroyed. I agree the energy has to something; after all, it holds the little particles of the body together. Is the energy aura, soul, or what? Is it not semantics here.

Sieglinde

Yes, but does it not make sense that it could be the same electromagnetic frequency that we came into the illusion of a body with. Program is program. Here or there, or is it always present at the same time? Birth and death may be the made-up semantics.

Dr. Ongley

Suppose I give you 10X vision and you see me enlarged. Then I give you 100X vision and you look at the same little spot. Then I give you 1000X vision—now, are you going to see more space or subspace?

Sieglinde

I won't see you at all.

Dr. Ongley

Right. So what holds the bits, whatever they call them? Let's say these bits give you the shape of a toe for example. The obvious answer is the electromagnetic force. This holds it together. Even if we were talking about atoms, there is more space that substance. So if you release that energy correctly of course we know what happens. You can have atomic fission if it's released that way. Is this within your body, the hydrogen bomb?

Sieglinde

We are back to semantics. The potential is probably there, only it shows up as an explosion in the body. Example, a stroke or a heart attack, et cetera. We do go off. It shows up verbally, mentally, or physically as a breakdown. Is it a possibility that persons are drawn to drugs too numb and prolong this explosion even if it amounts to death?

. . .

Let's get back to the body and how we can prevent the explosion and have optimal health.

Dr. Ongley

Oh, now you're talking treatments. If indeed what's holding us together is an electromagnetic force, isn't that what we should talk about? The Chinese talk about the flow of chi. What impedes the flow of chi? Mechanical problems. If you have a dislocated knee, the chi cant flow. For thousands of years this has been common knowledge. In the United States many refer to the human as a walking garbage can with the polluted air, fast food, stress, anger, et cetera. The Chinese would simply say you have impeded the flow of chi.

People in the health field today might say the individual cell can't function properly because it is filled with the toxins of nicotine, alcohol, drugs, white sugar. The cell can't do its job. In a broader sense, let's look at the liver. The bile is stored in the gallbladder. When you eat, out it goes to help you and your digestion. This is the gallbladder composed of millions of cells. Now take it down to the individual cell. If there is a blockage in the bile duct, the bile can't flow down to process the food. How do you get the toxins out of the impeding cells?

Sieglinde

You can do Tai Chi, jump on a trampoline to move things out of the lymph system, exercise the mind to think happy and grateful thoughts. I'm sure there are many possibilities. I think being happy may be our biggest cure and to see new adventures on the horizon to look forward to.

. . .

Dr. Ongley

There are people who sit in an electromagnetic hoop and try to change the electromagnetic field to normalize things. If you go to China and watch them do Tai Chi, do they have less sickness and live longer? Evaluate the results. The basic rule here is to test anything by their results. Even in China, people are confused about the overall problem as we are. Leave out the mysticism of India and China and look at the results. I saw on the news there is some dear lady in the United States who is the oldest woman in the world—118 years old. Run along to her and ask her if she practiced Tai Chi.

Sieglinde

She probably worked her entire life and never thought about her age and did not celebrate birthdays, only her newfound wisdom along the way. She loved what she did and had a reason to wake up every morning and generally loved life.

Dr. Ongley

Now isn't that wonderful? We are right back to square one. She did what she did when she wanted and harmed no one. A basic principle.

Let's take what I would classify the unknown garbage. I've been over that wall. What I learned on the other side of the wall is the elixir of life. That's why Ulysses got on his boat to go out and find these things and he came back without them. In Columbus' day, oh my God, all of the trouble and it didn't work. Why doesn't it work? When you travel eight or ten thousand miles, you come to a different way of life, a different everything. Actually nothing has changed.

. . .

Sieglinde

True. I just want to add that we all know that Columbus did not discover America; he was simply sent to conquer it.

Now, why do we have cancer, heart disease, et cetera?

Dr. Ongley

Because we want it. Let's face the facts: How do we know anything but by the results? You want it. It is a choice, be it unconscious. Take 100 people who don't have AIDS. Tell them what causes it and tell them to stay away from that. When they get AIDS, they choose it. It's that simple.

The message I am trying to give you is that nothing has changed. People have had long, lingering deaths throughout history, or you can go into a hospital and be dead three days later. Nothing has changed. Let us assume that the traveler who comes home brings with him the elixir of life and the human will never accept that he has the secret. You must go to the mountains of Tibet and run through the mountains of China. The Chinese could say, "I'll go to the United States and run up and down Mt. McKinley then I'll have the secret."

Let's look at Kung Fu movies and let's look at the acting here. The whole object of the movie was to get the book of knowledge and everyone who went off got slain by a monkey or a dragon. One fellow finally made it and he rushed up and found the book. It was completely blank. And there was the fellow who preceded him and just kept smiling. We are seeking something which isn't there.

. . .

Sieglinde

I see the same smile on your face most all the time. Through it all, you know the secret and you are living it and are willing to pay the price for being here and doing your work. No matter what.

When we speak of what the future has in store for all of us, I must share an experience that I had in the clinic on the beautiful Island of St. Maarten in the Caribbean. What a great place for us to spend time while I am recording your wisdom. The people here have a gentle grace and a knowing which hopefully will carry many of us into the future.

The sky was wet and heavy with rain; it had poured and a river was hitting the front wheel of my rental car parked in front of the clinic. While waiting for Dr. Abadjief, the receptionist Meta had served me coffee and we chatted while the rain poured all around her living area. The walls are open at all times so the Caribbean breezes gently drift through the home. Waiting for my treatment, I went back out into the waiting area when an elderly black woman came in with a yellow T-shirt, a turban wrapped around her head with a matching wrap around a long dress, very colorful and handsome on this tall and gracious woman. Her voice was gentle and her eyes smiled with light. Her red sandals were in her hand and she was barefoot. She was soaked.

She had some questions about her bill, which turned out to be no problem. Meta crumpled it up and tossed it into a large webbed metal wastebasket. They smiled and exchanged a few words. I joined in for a moment when this lovely woman turned around to me with a huge smile looking at the tornado-like rain outside. She told me that in her next life, "I think I will be a duck," with a giggle. We all smiled and I said jokingly, "Why not a beautiful swan?" She said, looking into my eyes with her voice lowered, "A duck is every bit as happy as a swan." The simple beauty of that sent shivers through me as if I had experience divinity or God. I felt as if I knew nothing and asked, "What is the mystery I find here?"

Dr. Ongley

I don't know yet but I see and hear this from people every day in the world, and yes there is something very special here. It lives in the heart of the people.

Sieglinde

This was 1990. In 1991 I was here when the big hurricane came and completely destroyed this island for several years. Dr. Ongley and I were the last two people who got on the last plane out and the hurricane followed us to Puerto Rico and then on to Miami. I felt very sad for the people but I am sure they took it with grace and much humbleness.

It is now many, many years later. We have talked about taking responsibility for our health and our bodies. How can we best understand what the messages are since, buy the result, we create our conditions? When we dream and study our dreams, we learn what the different symbols mean. Does the body, when it is out of balance and diseased, speak to us in a similar language?

Dr. Ongley

I think the answer to that is yes. The whole thought that we are suggesting is where the patient feels the pain is a clue to the doctor, of the origin of the source. Where is the source of that pain? So we had a definition of referred pain, pain felt elsewhere than at its source. When the patient is describing to the physician where he or she happens to feel pain, the doctor should be thinking, *Gee, I know where the pain is coming from.* Now it might come from more than one little spot or it's possible that the pain is coming from several spots. His job should be to introduce local anesthetic into one of the places that could possibly be causing the pain. If the pain goes away, he has made a precise diagnosis and this is a tremendous advantage of the work done by people like Sir Thomas Lewis on referred pain.

Charts subsequently made by Lewis, Calgrin, Steinberg and all the others are all hanging up on their walls as the patient who is describing the pain. The doctor would say, "Oh when Calgrin injected spot A, it precipitated a pain running down the specific part of the limb."

We have many common examples in medicine. Even when I was in medical school, you must be very careful when a patient comes in rubbing the front of her thigh just above the knee. You don't immediately rush down and examine the knee because most commonly her pain is coming from her hip. Many physicians will spend hours and hours examining and looking at the knee and finding it perfectly normal because he has forgotten that most commonly the hip refers pain to the knee, as the lower back refers pain to the hip. Worse still when we are dealing with referred pain there are many things that alter the distance and the intensity of the referred pain. The more deeper structures do not refer pain as accurately. Through clinical examination he should be testing the various structures and when he discovers the structure which is causing the pain, infiltrate it with a local anesthetic—and again, if the pain goes away, he made the diagnosis.

Sieglinde

Can all patients identify specifically where the pain is?

Dr. Ongley

Two out of ten cannot.

Sieglinde

How can we identify our own pain? I imagine the doctor must develop highly developed probing skills for the truth of the condition to surface in the patient's own mind. When they say, "I hurt all over," this is very unlikely.

Dr. Ongley

This is why it is of paramount importance that the physician take a very detailed accurate history of the patient's complaint.

Sieglinde

It sounds like this falls into the previously mentioned category of boredom for the doctor.

Dr. Ongley

For most doctors, yes. It should be thought of as a detective mystery. He is trying to sift it all out and figure out mechanically. If it is mechanical, where is this pain emanating from? What exactly is the problem?

. . .

Sieglinde

What he really needs to do then is facilitate the patient sifting out the problem so he can solve the mystery himself by isolating the mystery of the pain.

Dr. Ongley

Lots of famous physicians have used words like, "Patience, Doctor." The patient is telling you what is wrong. Listen. Don't tell the patient. You listen and ask questions. It is very important to find out if the pain came on suddenly. If we are talking of the musculoskeletal system suddenly implies there was a traumatic event precipitated by movement that something tore. If something tore, good grief it probably bled. If it bled, the ramifications of bleeding inside a tissue as a part of the human frame is tremendous pain.

Sieglinde

My father fell, hurt his back, he couldn't sit, was eating laying on the floor and crawled down the sidewalk in south San Francisco for therapy every other day for weeks and was told the tests are all normal. "There is nothing wrong with you." My father was a very active man, walked a good eight miles per day. Never an ounce over-weight, ate only home-cooked meals. Never drank or smoked. In his youth he was a boxer and master in the art of karate. He was of a positive mindset. He was always singing and whistling and very active socially and in sports. He believed he would live to be 100 and was never sick.

Dr. Ongley

What they should have said is, "We can't find what's wrong with you." There is this confusion in medicine that says if they can't find anything then there is nothing wrong. My God, I can't figure this out because it is not normal for a person to have to crawl up and down a sidewalk, now is it? You said your father was very fit and healthy so he either became suddenly insane or he *didn't* become insane. If he became insane, his insanity was precipitated by a fall—which is not likely—but when he fell he injured something that simply didn't show up in the particular tests given by the physicians. He should have probed further, listened carefully, "What causes your pain?" If I wiggle my big toe it hurts me or it doesn't hurt me. If I wiggle my knee it hurts me or it doesn't, the hip and the back, et cetera.

There are certain movements in the back or the big toe that hurt when the patient moves them. Those structures are either being stretched or squeezed—so it should be perfectly logical, again, if half of the body is made up of ten separate structures it's very important that one is okay, two is okay, three is okay, number four is not okay... So the negatives are as important as the positives.

Sieglinde

So it's a matter of elimination as long as the diagnosis is thorough.

Dr. Ongley

Identification, not elimination. We are siting a perfect example of how we fail. Today in the office we were listening together of confessions of absolute failure. A girl with back problems was told by her physician to lie in bed for two months, don't move. What is this supposed to do? I understand back in the days of tubercular infection of the lung, the more the lung pumps in and out, the more it spreads and the bigger the lump of scar tissue that forms. Lie in bed and don't move and if you could save them, tell them not to breathe. Or put a lung to rest. But when it comes to the musculoskeletal system, what happens if you lie in bed two months?

Sieglinde

I would think the muscles get weak and the joints get stiff. The patient gets worse.

Dr. Ongley

There was a British physician who wrote a book entitled *The Dangers of Going to Bed*. It's very true. You get demineralization of bones and muscles, ligaments and all of those things. So from the point of view, yes the patient is made worse. If it is put to rest so the nature can heal, it makes some sense, but you have to weigh it up. Will it heal at rest or will it heal with certain activities? At rest we have these side effects and if it's going to heal up with certain activities he's better to heal up with activity. That is one of the principles I have been preaching for many years. Healing in the presence of movement.

Sieglinde

I hear this patient say that she is most comfortable when she is walking long distances yet the doctor said, "Go to bed for two months and don't move, and in a year you might get better."

Dr. Ongley

What is that based on, I wonder? In the meantime, you've lost a year of your life, a year of employment and feeling depressed and worthless.

Sieglinde

If the doctor had asked the right questions and she had said, "But I feel better when I walk long distances," which she did, what should he have done differently?

Dr. Ongley

This is what happens with many cardiac patients. They say to the doctor, "Look, you know you tell me to lay in bed and I feel worse so I started some physical exercises in the bed and I felt better and when you listened to my heart you said, 'Wow, it's stronger.' If I had listened to you and stayed in bed deteriorating, I would have been much worse. Now I have experienced healing with movement."

Sieglinde

Are you saying the body intuitively knows how to heal itself?

Dr. Ongley

Yes I am.

Sieglinde

How can we teach people this? How can they get in touch with this intuitive process that we are all born with?

Dr. Ongley

Let's get back to the girl patient. She was telling her doctor and he was not listening. Listen here, Doctor, the patient is telling you what is wrong. The patient may not have learned your particular language that you learned in medical school but she is telling you walking makes her better and you are telling her, "Don't do that. Do instead what makes you worse—lie in bed for two months." She said she feels worse laying down. Why is it that physicians don't listen? Why can't a patient contribute to her own healing? Tell the doctor, "I want you to listen to me. I am not just a patient who doesn't know what she is talking about. I'm giving you clues for my treatment."

Sieglinde

I can understand the confusion of the doctor. He must choose between what he has learned in a textbook, the medical bible, what his colleagues are doing, and what a layperson is saying.

Dr. Ongley

That's not necessarily the case. Let's take your father who fell down, shall we say. He felt something snap or tear. This had to cause bleeding and we know that if it bled, the clot forms scar tissue so you have two structures, one sort of at an angle to the other. Adhesions now bind the two together and when you move in either direction it pulls on the adhesions and it is very painful. It will probably rip away and bleed again. So it goes on and on. When you have moving parts and it comes to soft tissue, you have to have healing and it's unrealistic to assume that disc disintegrated. This takes time for them to disintegrate. If you are young and damage a disc let's say in an automobile accident, nothing shows on an x-ray for five years. In the time all discs disintegrate and that's why we lose a percentage of the length of our spine with age. So it it's a normal process for the discs to disintegrate. Why should we worry so much about a disintegrated disc?

By the time a child begins to walk, the nerve supply disappears. So a disc doesn't have a nerve supply. The only nerve supply that you have is just at the back portion, a bit of fibrous fatty supply so it can't hurt you.

Sieglinde

Why are we born with it then lose it?

Dr. Ongley

Probably from the healing in the presence of movement when the child starts to walk or grow. As you are growing and forming, you need to have, let us say, messengers coming to the top of the head.

Sieglinde

Might this not explain a child coming into the world knowing and remembering all and then beginning his process of forgetting the "all"?

Dr. Ongley

It does explain that if you interrupt the nerve supply to the muscles controlling the elbow joint and you can't move the elbow correctly than it fades away. So the converse is probably true. It requires an intact nerve supply in order to grow.

. . .

Sieglinde

So is it possible to get the nerve supply back that we lose as a small child beginning to walk?

Dr. Ongley

This is a question I ask many doctors. If a disc is devoid of blood supply, how on earth does a baby's disc grow up to be a big man's disc. There has to be another mechanism for the attrition to the disc.

Sieglinde

What is it?

Dr. Ongley

Well, the piece of lining of the vertical body in a joint is lined with articular cartilage. So we have bone, articular cartilage, and your disc, and below you have cartilage and the bone. The articular cartilage has many, many micro pores in it, and when you pound up and down you squeeze the nutrition from the bone above through the articular cartilage to the disc. Movement is absolutely essential. If you can't have movement, you can't

have the nutrition. So again, if we talk about the articular cartilage which lines the head of your femur and lines the cavity of the acetabulum and it doesn't have blood supply, how does the little man's hip joint grow into the big man's hip joint? So now you understand.

If the normal nutrition to a cervical joint depends upon a pressure effect, and you tell someone who has degenerative arthritis the more you use it the sooner you'll wear it out. "Lie around in bed all day." The reverse is true. Think of the millions of people who have been harmed because we gave them the wrong treatment. None of we physicians take the responsibility because we did what was written in a textbook, which was based upon nothing.

Sieglinde

The patient also doesn't want to go through the pain of the movement. They would rather take a pill.

Dr. Ongley

I understand this so isn't it much better to give them a pill and give them movement. To give them a pill and lie them in bed—that is a serious crime.

I mentioned the loss of the nervous supply in the baby to you because there are many changes in the body of course, but most of the structures of the body are blessed with having this nervous supply. I mentioned to you that discs don't and articular cartilage don't have this nervous supply.

Sieglinde

In orthopedic medicine, what are the most common ailments?

Dr. Ongley

Pain is the most common. Of pain in general, the most common pain in general is of the musculoskeletal system. In this system it's probably a toss-up between neck and back pain.

. . .

Sieglinde

Is everything in the body linked to the spine?

Dr. Ongley

Obviously your legs are linked to the back, so what are you asking me?

Sieglinde

The chiropractor, for example, believes that every portion of the spine sends messages to and is related to all organs and most all functions of the body. What is your opinion about this?

Dr. Ongley

This is where the chiropractor leads you astray. Remember, we must go back. There must be something awry within a tissue of the body—either it is twisted or damaged in some way and then all of the little nerve endings are triggered or there is a chemical imbalance in the area of the structures that trigger the nerve receptors, the nerve endings. So it's either traumatic or chemical.

Sieglinde

If there is a chemical imbalance in the pancreas, can that show up or does it come from a particular part of the spine? The charts in the chiropractor's office imply this.

Dr. Ongley

The chiropractor tends to lead you to believe that you have a malplacement in your spine which causes every condition. Now you have to have a malplacement in your spine to get AIDS. Does that make sense?

Sieglinde

That's an interesting example. And seems drastic.

Dr. Ongley

Why? Before the AIDS epidemic, I used to say another word before I can get venereal disease, syphilis, gonorrhea, et cetera. I must have a malplacement in my spine. Mr. Chiropractor, you can straighten my spine and I will immediately have sex with a woman who has venereal disease and I won't catch it.

Sieglinde

Isn't that an accurate example?

Dr. Ongley

It's an accurate example, yes. The whole thing is absolute nonsense. You have to have a malplacement in your spine to catch a disease? This is what the chiropractor and his charts are saying to you.

Sieglinde

I've never seen a little line coming from the spine on a chart that points to something in the body called AIDS.

Dr. Ongley

Of course that knocks it into a cock hat, doesn't it? But they show you all of the little nervous connections to the organs and I say, "Fine. If the spine is not pushing on the nerve, for example, let's talk about the penis then. I can't get gonorrhea." It's utter nonsense. I can get gonorrhea with or without a displacement pushing on the nerves on the spine which innovates the penis. Did Louis Pasteur live and die in vain? Do you have to have malplacement in the spine to have disease or you have bugs doing it?

Sieglinde

I'm amazed. I've always thought the organ's function was directly connected to the spine. It takes a drastic example like yours to get it. I can't begin to imagine all of the medical misinformation that the masses of people believe to be the truth.

Dr. Ongley

A tremendous amount. But you use the example that I have given you because it is so common and simple to say to the chiropractor that you can get AIDS without having a malplacement of the spine. He will blush. So if you can get AIDS, how many other conditions can you get and suffer from? Now explain to me if I have AIDS how manipulating the spine is going to help me.

Sieglinde

Then how does manipulating, cracking, and stretching the spine help anyone?

Dr. Ongley

Let's finish with this theory. If I have AIDS and you manipulate my spine, are you going to cure me?

. . .

Sieglinde

AIDS is an immune problem and an extreme example.

Dr. Ongley

Yes, but let's backtrack now. When does it begin to apply that by manipulating the spine, something in the body is cured? Let's take diabetes. Is diabetes due to a malplacement of the spine?

Sieglinde

No.

Dr. Ongley

But it's on the chart. You've seen it on the chart. If you are going to talk about nebulous things like irritated bowels, constipation...chiropractors go on and on about this and they are all on the chart.

Sieglinde

There is nothing on the chart about hypoglycemia.

Dr. Ongley

Chiropractors are now starting to talk about it and they are manipulating you for it. You see, now you get down to the next facet. If you have a dislocated shoulder, structures must be stretched or torn to allow the joint to dislocate. It cannot dislocate if something isn't stretched or torn. So to have the malplacement, you have to have a structure which is stretched or torn. It's over here out of place. You put it back with some form of manipulation. What's going to keep it there?

. . .

Sieglinde
Nothing.

Dr. Ongley
The chiropractor will say, "Oh your muscles will do that." The muscles can't do it because all a muscles does is move a joint. It doesn't hold it in place, it moves it. The things that hold joints in place, synovial joints, in particular are ligaments.

So it is the same as the unstable knee. You think if you continuously manipulate an unstable knee, it will become stable. Then you have 50,000 people who will say, "I don't believe that because I had a pain in my back and I went to fifty-four MDs and they couldn't help me and I went to the chiropractor and he went *click* and I was cured." So if the patient just went to the chiropractor and never to the MDs, then the chiropractors would be manipulating cancer and spinal tumors et cetera, which by the way he does. With, by the way, devastating effects on the patient.

The best answer is to take the health professionals and call him willy nilly whatever you like and add to his training these different facets like manipulation.

Sieglinde
Again, how can people educate themselves?

Dr. Ongley

By reading your book. Once it's published it will be taken up by health editors all around the world and they will take parts of it and write articles about it and the public will read small facets and let's get rid of this discogenic theory of the causation of all neck and back pain but in a very, very minor percentage.

Sieglinde

What do you do with pain that is not physical but manifests itself in the body?

Dr. Ongley

All pain has an origin. Either mechanics or chemistry. Or it is purely emotional. If it is the latter, the patient needs to go to a professional who deals with emotional pain.

Sieglinde

Is it not difficult for the patient to know when the physician is not asking the right questions?

Dr. Ongley

Not if he wants to determine if the pain is a truly deferred pain or a pain radiating down a nerve and he can then determine if there is a legitimate basis for the pain, take out his bottle of local anesthetic and simply give an injection into the area and if the patient says, "Wow, it's gone!" then he is true blue.

Sieglinde

And if the pain is still there?

. . .

Dr. Ongley

Then you have to assume it is on the emotional level. Most discomfort does have its basis in the emotion. I don't profess to be a psychiatrist.

Sieglinde

Many people suffer from depression, is that not an emotional state that can manifest as pain?

Dr. Ongley

Depression does not necessarily cause pain. Depression makes you depressed. You can have a depressed person and ask them if they are in pain. If they have pain it is made worse by the emotional state. Depression as such does not cause pain.

Sieglinde

What people really should want to hear is how important their emotional state is when dealing with pain.

Dr. Ongley

Yes. You can have two people coming in with a compound fracture of the leg. One person comes in screaming in agony and the other person comes in and says, "I busted my leg." Why the difference? It is the emotional aspect of pain. Now again let us emphasize over and over again, we are not saying that a person who has severe pain is precipitating it inside their heads. We are not saying that. What we are saying is that the emotional center has a tremendous effect on pain.

. . .

Sieglinde

If a person is in a fragile emotional state, does it increase the pain trifold or more?

Dr. Ongley

Even more.

Sieglinde

Let's say someone just went through a divorce.

Dr. Ongley

Now you are so happy to have gotten rid of that so and so of a wife and you cut your finger, it doesn't hurt at all.

Sieglinde

Very great.

Dr. Ongley

See where your mind is, I fooled you. You are always thinking on the other side of it. You cannot assume just because you have gone through a divorce that you are unhappy.

Sieglinde

There seems to be so much drama around divorce these days even though it is an everyday occurrence. In the US, 2.5 out of 3 marriages end in divorce. Every magazine you pick up, it is always telling people what the most ninety-eight traumatic experiences in life are. The first is a death, then divorce, loss of work et cetera. So these are all negative connotations to the experience.

Dr. Ongley

And I disagree. You see, I have talked to many people who are absolutely elated to finally be divorced. "I am off to marry Louise or John."

Sieglinde

This is merely replacement and the same issues will crop up because we are the problem in most cases and not the other person. We have now learned nothing and wasted much time and precious life force.

Dr. Ongley

It doesn't matter—it's still divorce, isn't it?

Sieglinde

There is a little difference having your teeth pulled out today and running around toothless as compared to having a new shiny set put in the same day.

Dr. Ongley

We are not talking about teeth. We are talking about divorce. Oprah was doing her show on TV the other night. People said, "Hey, I want to get rid of this guy; it is not working anymore. It's not what I expected." Now you give that woman who is making that statement the money, the house, and the car. She is going to be depressed? I don't think so. No way. The guy will be. She will be elated.

Sieglinde

Then she will probably find a guy just like the first one and go through the same thing all over again. Maybe even add to her lifestyle.

Dr. Ongley

Exactly. We understand that people gravitate back to sameness. You cannot tell that to people. You cannot tell them they are causing their own misery.

Sieglinde

Why not? I do when they come to me for support.

Dr. Ongley

You can, but they don't want to hear that, so what is the point?

Sieglinde

My sweet Dr. Ongley, you are so frustrating. Like a dog with a bone you don't let it go. Much laughter and a tea break now. Speaking to people's ability to hear is quite an art form.

Dr. Ongley

When they are ready to have a different experience they will, but it is not because you told them. I saw a patient this morning. I saw her the other day and her husband was there and their child was there. I had to make up my mind the other day that no matter what I said, this woman could not hear me. The husband heard, as did the child, but she did not. The next day she asked me all of the same questions and several times I had to say to her, "This is what you just asked me." She was not hearing me at all. She had some idea in her head which is characteristic of humans that the idea in their head is supposed to bear fruit for them. And when you tell them over and over again that idea is not going to work no matter how you phrase the response, whatever I tell her of the situation she does not hear it. They do not like your answer. I finally said, "You just don't like the answer I'm giving you."

Sieglinde

This is true—people want to be told what they want to hear. Sad, really.

Dr. Ongley

That's it.

Sieglinde

How do you communicate with a mass of people on a level that all can understand and comprehend? Our minds are programmed and filled with what advertisers, politicians, doctors, the media want us to believe. What other way have powerful leaders throughout history done this?

Dr. Ongley

Every writer in the field of medicine is told that the intelligence of people is that of an eleven- or twelve-year-old. You must make it diabolically simple.

. . .

Sieglinde

Yet there is great complexity in books and scientific research.

Dr. Ongley

The books are not best sellers and the research is mostly read by other researchers and professionals in the field.

You ask me how to get the message across to the average person. You make it simple, precise, and clear. Now back it up with scientific proof. People are not stupid. They are hungry for the truth; very few people are willing to tell it like it is. With example after example, people can test themselves and come to their own conclusions. I tell doctors all the time, "You push on your ulnar nerve on your elbow and you are aware of a bit of discomfort. You have a feeling of pins and needles in your fingers at the distal end." So when someone gets pressure on a nerve trunk, they should be feeling it down in the foot or wherever. Not in the elbow. You can do this on yourself. How come when you go into a doctor's office the doctor doesn't know that?

Sieglinde

Most people are told that if their hands and feet are cold, it must be a circulation problem. This is not always the case then.

Dr. Ongley

Right, this is not always true. It can be a myriad of things. If there is anemia, he would have cold hands and feet. If there was pressure on the spinal cord, he would have cold hands and feet.

. . .

Sieglinde

What is the myth about migraine headaches?

Dr. Ongley

What is migraine? It is a severe headache. There are many causes of severe headaches. Let's take, for example, a tumor in the brain. It will give you a severe headache. Is that a migraine? You fall and smack the back of your head, you get a severe headache. Is that a migraine? Or there is a clinical entity where you get half a headache preceded by an aura where on premonition you see different-colored lights. A different type of aura, Sieglinde, from the one you are smiling about. You become hypersensitive to light, noise and sometimes you vomit. I can inject an irritant into certain parts of the upper cervical spine in the base of the skull that will precipitate those things. And this has nothing to do with blood vessels expanding in the brain.

Many people go raving on about something they heard from a doctor and believe it to be the gospel truth. So the converse can happen—the patient can come in and describe all of those things and you find the areas that can refer the pain and the symptoms that accompany it. You can now take care of that patient rather simply. The majority of headaches can be helped or taken care of, but don't tell the headache society of America this. Again, harkening back to the woman who was talking to me this morning and wanting a guarantee. I said, "Guarantee what, that I'll be living and breathing tomorrow? That you as a patient will be here tomorrow on time? Can you guarantee that?" There are a multiplicity of pains in different areas. You fix one and you might not fix the others. "Oh, my arm still hurts me, you didn't cure me." The guarantee is null and void. How stupid can you get? This is not—and I repeat, *not*—an example of a patient taking responsibility for her health.

Sieglinde

Obviously, this person is not taking personal responsibility, most likely not in any area of her life. Assuming a person is a normal rational human being with a multitude of pains, she may get very frustrated and angry when help is not received everywhere instantly.

Dr. Ongley

And how many normal rational people do we have? Psychiatrists will tell you that two out of ten will be relatively normal at that point in time.

Sieglinde

Interesting. What is relatively normal through the eyes of a psychiatrist? Studies show we live on a planet of mass neurosis.

Dr. Ongley

Yes. Not neurotic, simply abnormal. Relatively normal and there are times when those relatively normal people will have bits or bouts of insanity due to anger, frustration, jealousy, vengeance, et cetera. Then you go on to frustration and it *is* frustrating for a patient to go from doctor to doctor to doctor and finally be labeled a neurotic because the doctors won't take the time or don't have the knowledge to sit down and figure out what is the problem. Or they just don't care.

. . .

It is interesting to note here that the written rule is, never give a pain-relieving medication to the undiagnosed abdomen. Everyone in medicine knows this. If the doctor does not have a definite diagnosis, for example appendicitis, and he gives the patient pain-relieving medication, that appendix can swell and burst. The patient is now measurably worse off because he doesn't feel it since he is filled with narcotics. This is the written rule again: Do not ever give narcotics to the undiagnosed abdomen. Why shouldn't that rule be applied to the rest of the body, the back or the shoulder? If you haven't got a precise diagnosis of the shoulder and back then you should not give pain-relieving medications. The same logic holds.

Sieglinde

There are many doctors who will prescribe whatever the patient wants. TV commercials tell you ask your doctors for this if you have this symptom and people actually do this.

Dr. Ongley

We are not saying the medical profession is filled with gallant knights. It is filled with human beings. He tries his best; he is only human. Too few pat him on the back when he is right and everyone attacks him when he is wrong. This is human and happens in all areas of life. Judge your doctor as you would judge yourself.

Sieglinde

But we don't judge ourselves.

Dr. Ongley

No not at all, so again we are talking about two sets of rules.

One for me and another for you. Unfortunately within the medical profession, the doctor has a set of rules for him and another set of rules for the patient.

Going back to another patient today who wasn't really calling for a second opinion (which is eminently reasonable). She was asking a doctor to look at everything that I did but didn't want me to look at everything that he did. Now if it was a second opinion and this chappy is overseas in the United States, how on earth can you get a second opinion over the telephone? This is absolute nonsense. When this is pointed out, it becomes apparent that this individual patient is simply trying to lead you astray for a reason which is so ridiculous it makes me laugh. And the reason behind it all for her was that she was afraid of injections. All she had say was, "I am in agony and want you to help me because I was referred here and know that you can help me. Yet I am terrified of injections." Why rush around the mulberry bush fifty-five times and not face the problem? Everyone is afraid to seek the truth. As Jack Nicholson so humbly stated, "You can't handle the truth."

Sieglinde

You are advising people, then, to take responsibility for themselves by demanding the truth. "Doctor, can you fix my neck?" If he can't, he becomes a false prophet. A patient must be a truth seeker. This may be difficult to answer for the doctor and to be willing to tell the truth.

Dr. Ongley

They simply can't. Lord Horder, who was twice president of the British Medical Association, said of the medical profession in general—and this is why he did have a third term—"We help ten percent, we kill ten percent, and the other eighty percent heal themselves." So again, if that be the truth, can you face that in a medical profession? So again, if you have a heart problem go to the heart specialist, "Can you cure my heart?" He says no. You have a liver problem and go to the liver man and he says, "No, I can't." You have lung cancer and you go to the cancer specialist and ask, "Can you cure my cancer?" and he says no. How can you be a prophet? In the days before antibiotics, what did doctors care? Do you think in those days the doctors were treated any less like a god as they are today? But they have cured nothing.

Sieglinde

Don't people always want heroes and want to believe what they want to believe?

Dr. Ongley

So take George Washington, the father of the United States, on his deathbed being bled, and bled again. He said, "Oh God, protect me from my doctors." So he was finally bled out and died. I've mentioned to you many times the wonderful institution in Los Angeles Cedars-Sinai Hospital and I mentioned to you Lucille Ball, she didn't come out; Danny Kaye, he didn't come out; and the countless number of others who followed, never came out alive. How come if they have the very best of medicine together within those walls, why don't people come out alive?

Sieglinde

Now wait a minute. There is a time clock ticking for each of us when it is time for us to die.

. . .

Dr. Ongley

Okay, then why put them in the hospital? We are not debating that it's their time to die. I am asking, why put them in the hospital with all of the expenses and additional suffering? Why doesn't the doctor look them in the eye and say, "You're going to die, wouldn't you be happier in your own bed in a familiar environment with your friends and loved ones?" Oh no, we will go to the hospital. A tremendous expense, with this person doing this and the other one doing another thing and on and on we go. Now either the medical profession is trying to save him or they are hoodwinking themselves and the patient.

Sieglinde

I am very clear that medicine does not want to get into the mystery of death and the natural dying process that the body has been through so often it has become a habit, and consistently the same. But dying with dignity and grace should be respected and encouraged in the medical community.

Dr. Ongley

Oh heavens no. It would be nice, however. I know you don't like the word *scientific*, we mentioned that before, but let us seek the truth. My definition again of scientific is current knowledge. So black is black today, then we get more knowledge and find out that that black is white in the exact reverse.

Sieglinde

But you still have a dozen different interpretations.

Dr. Ongley

That's not the point. Scientific laypeople and physicians believe that scientific means fact.

Sieglinde

But it does not.

Dr. Ongley

Of course it doesn't, it couldn't possibly. It simply means today's fact is wrong tomorrow. If you go to a court of law, whatever that court finds is fact. It doesn't matter if it's right or wrong; it is now fact.

Sieglinde

Yet the definition of truth is real things, events, and facts. Yet truth seems selective.

Dr. Ongley

People don't like the truth and they don't want to hear it. If you suddenly took out a shotgun and said, "You better disagree." Very quickly a light comes on. An example is one of these rape cases, he says, "Oh but I couldn't help it, it wasn't my fault." Oh really? With the double barrels in your mouth, buster, now you can help it? It all depends on the circumstances whether you can help it or not. The circumstances change and the results change.

Sieglinde

The truth is a big subject. I have heard it said, "First the truth will always piss you off."

. . .

Dr. Ongley

Yes. Many people have been fed shun fables. It is very difficult to tell people there is no Santa Claus. They have been programmed their entire life that doctors know best and are correct. He is not necessarily correct. All we are doing is suggesting to choose a doctor and know that there may be another alternative, not that he is wrong all the time. We are not suggesting that, in certain cases, there may be an alternative approach.

Sieglinde

How can we expect people to be open to other options when they don't take responsibility for health? They want a quick artificial fix. They aren't even willing to do what it takes to get out of a job they hate and begin something new.

Dr. Ongley

People are very willing if there is a reward in it for them. You suddenly say to a person, "Here is a suitcase with ten million dollars —it's yours." Suddenly they accept an alternative because they want to.

Sieglinde

So the question is what is your life and health worth?

Dr. Ongley

Yes. Is your back worth ten million dollars, for example? Now, we have another problem and a big question. Do you really want to be healthy? People ask me all the time about particular therapies, you know. Do they have side effects. I say, "Yes, the side effect is that you will get well." For some, the drama and attention, the love from being sick is more important.

Sieglinde

This is true in my opinion.

Dr. Ongley

We have talked about bedrest and things like that. Your body is much more intricately attuned than the world's best Rolls Royce automobile. You say, "I've got a Rolls Royce at home but it doesn't work so I leave it in the garage." So I have a Rolls Royce for a back and I put it in the bed and leave it there. It's stupid.

Both are of the best craftsmanship. It's a marvelous car but it doesn't run. Your back is not functioning as it is supposed to, so does it make any more sense to lay it in the bed than to keep the broken Rolls in the garage because maybe some little thing isn't working?

Sieglinde

Maybe the difference is the back is built to function perfectly and a car is built to fall apart. There is more money in parts. Isn't it also interesting how much money there is in keeping people in physical distress?

Dr. Ongley

Now I don't want to throw those rocks. In medicine we are not only dealing with the horrible money thing, the economics, but the ego of the participants—the doctor and the patient.

. . .

Sieglinde

People seem to be attracted to holistic care thinking they are treating the entire body.

Dr. Ongley

I've spent my lifetime working to study one particular facet of the human body and I certainly haven't learned it all. It would be beyond my capabilities to do the entirety of the human body. One person may have the capability of realizing that he doesn't know one particular facet of the medical approach to the human body, therefore he sends that patient to the appropriate specialist. But I don't see that happening. I see the one individual attempting to take care of all the different aspects of medicine to the detriment of the patient.

Sieglinde

So it might take twenty doctors to make a person optimally well.

Dr. Ongley

We are all taught a screening process through your history and a physical examination. So from the point of view, the whole person should always have been paramount in the doctor's approach. He should have realized that if his forte is in the chest, and if the patient's symptoms indicate a liver problem, the patient should be referred. In my day, growing up in medicine, that is what happened. I'm seeing particularly in the United States today they don't do extensive histories. Today you fill out a form with all of your history, et cetera, for the file but doctors don't really look at it. Physicals are beginning to leak into a form of treatment based on nutrition, were getting older, the anti-aging vogues, whether it be chelation therapy or everyone should take selenium or B12, whatever it happens to be. These things are talked about at the medical meetings and the doctor goes back to his office and says, "Well I haven't been doing that," so he gives it to all of his patients. The same type of treatment with a minor variation, but everyone seems to get the same. And we have mentioned the chiropractors, where everyone is getting manipulation.

The chiropractor today is jumping into what is being termed *holistic care* or *alternative medical care* and he is giving the patients everything. There seems to be no true indications and contra-indications for any particular therapy of the administration for medicines or drugs. We hear that the trauma field, particularly if it's minor, arnica is wonderful and everyone who comes in the door gets arnica. Arnica is a plant that grows on the mountainside in the Alps and it's been known for a long, long time that if you fall down the same mountain and you grab hold of the arnica plant and you chew it up, it prevents bruising and minor injuries, et cetera.

Then people jump on the bandwagon and everyone gets arnica. Today the different varieties of CBD tinctures are very popular and come in many forms—salves for muscle aches, and rubs for joints. They work quite well. Hospice patients are given this often instead of morphine to be alert and relieved before their transition. Selenium is another product in vogue so everyone gets their manipulation then runs to the health food store to get some but more than likely the chiropractor also sells it.

One of the ongoing contentions in the United States is that the medical profession is wanting to take over the health food stores. They use the excuse that they want to regulate, just as I am suggesting, true indications or contra-indications to anything you put inside your body. Just don't use it. The individual should know what is good for his body and what is bad for it. You shouldn't have to go to a doctor to find this out. You'll be told that bacon and eggs have so much cholesterol that if you eat bacon and eggs, you'll be dead in ten years. People can eat this for fifty years every day and nothing happens.

Sieglinde

Every day one hears of something else that causes cancer.

Dr. Ongley

Yes. As far as I'm concerned, anything in medicine—which has a multiplicity of treatments—indicates the medical profession has not found a treatment leading to the cure. We have mentioned throughout that simplicity seems to be the way to solve the complicated problem. It is complicated when you don't understand. When you understand it, the simple approach solves it.

Sieglinde

In talking about simple causes or simple approaches, aren't the greatest problems a form of disease or imbalance in the human body? Could it be that this imbalance is caused by negative emotions? Example, fear, blame, stress, shame, jealousy, anger, rage, victimhood, and so on?

Dr. Ongley

Now you are trying to lead me here. I maintain that from the days of Pasteur that bacteriologic origin of disease was accepted. Most people will agree that these things are in the body in a subclinical dose. Then something happens, and they multiply and start taking over the body and you get the manifestation of that particular disease, whether it is tuberculosis or influenza or what have you. What you are trying to get at is why is influenza, for example, which is in the body, in a subclinical way, why does it suddenly manifest itself in a clinical way when you have the symptoms of the eyes and the nose and whatever else goes with it?

Sieglinde

Is it not true that these people who think they are going to be sick are the ones most likely to manifest the disease?

Dr. Ongley

Now wait, let's slow down a little. If we are sitting here talking to Linus Pauling, he would say that stress depletes vitamin C in the body. The influenza is now able to take over and give you that condition. Now you will talk to another person who will say nebulous words like "It depletes the immune system." What does this actually mean, depletion of the immune system? Does the immune system go away? Does it disappear? What happens? Or does it mean that the function of the immune system is not adequate to cope with the problem at that particular time?

Sieglinde

If what you think about expands, and you say to me, "Only thinking makes it so," then it cannot be denied that there is a mental emotional influence.

. . .

Dr. Ongley

Many people will argue with physicians and claim it is mental; however, you have the problem if we are going to agree that bug A in the body is not normal, but it is there and it has been there for many years and suddenly causes a problem, how does it manifest itself? Is it because you are older? Is it because you ate too much sugar? Or is it because you read the book, *Sugar Blues*? Or what is it? If you read health magazines or read research on the internet in January, by the time you get to December everything they said in January is already outdated. In other words, no one knows the reason.

Sieglinde

So it must be an intangible, something other than what we have discussed and what science has labored over up until now. Or the truth is hidden from us by the powers to be on our planet.

Dr. Ongley

Correct.

Sieglinde

Is it possible that a germ, which we say is inside the body and is created there, is in fact outside the body and brought in through the six-foot electromagnetic energy field, especially when it is weak? Studies do confirm that the large field around us changes; for example, if you have a headache, the field is sucked in to support the area of the headache or wherever in the body we have a pain or injury. Also drugs will puncture holes in this field, allowing all sort of things floating around into our weaker bodies.

. . .

Dr. Ongley

We have been emphasizing there that bug A cannot be classified as a normal inhabitant of the body, and how did it get there, Sieglinde? Illness can be a great teacher. Is it possible that we pull it in at a time when we are weak, and like divine creators of our reality, we manifest illness whenever we need it for whatever reason that might be?

We are talking about droplets that are spread around, wingspread and various things—maybe we could have someone on an isolated island who suddenly comes down with a rare disease. How do you explain that?

Sieglinde

How does a person will himself to die? One morning I went to check on my mother and after an hour or so we were sitting in the living room and she said to me, "I am going to die today. Amanda (my six-year-old granddaughter who died exactly ten weeks prior in a car accident) can't wait for me any longer." I was in shock and speechless looking into my mother's eyes. She wanted to lay in bed and I lay with her. This was about noon. I held her hand we talked about all sorts of things she wanted to share.

When my mother was showing signs—I had seen many times doing hospice—of the body shutting down from the feet on up, as the colon shut down my mother willed herself with my help to the toilet to empty her bowels because she did not want a mess in the bed. At 8:30 she began to loudly speak in tongues to many people at the same time and I could not understand anything. An hour later she suddenly looked at me as I held her hand: "Don't be giving me any energy." I promised I would not do that. Around 9:30 she said, "This is not as easy as I thought."

She passed at 11:30 PM and I have never seen her as beautiful. No lines in her face, her legs showed no varicose veins. She glowed as if she was fluorescent. Her mouth was slightly open and a bubble formed with her last breath like those we blow into the air through the round end we dunk in the bottle of fluid. Her bubble even showed the same rainbow color. It remained there until I was able to call the funeral home for removal. How do we explain any of this?

Dr. Ongley

I think we understand that to a degree. Whatever it is within us that causes us to reproduce or to live has very essential facets to human nature. If you turn them off then you can create your death.

Sieglinde

If you can create a conscious death, then creating influenza must be child's play. I personally refuse to get a flu shot because of its detrimental contents and my belief that I won't get the flu is strong. I have not had the flu in twenty-five years.

Concerning death, it is my opinion and experience that there is a connection or a pull of some kind from persons on the other side of the veil who sometimes assist when the person is ready.

Dr. Ongley

People don't necessarily die of a disease. When the witch doctor says you are going to die and you happen to die, you don't die of a disease. What is causing the death?

Sieglinde

What difference does it make?

Dr. Ongley

It makes no difference. It is like the man who goes to bed at night and instead of waking up, he is dead.

Sieglinde

Is it not true that once a cancer patient is told he has cancer and to what degree, he becomes filled with doom and fear, and suddenly the cells spread faster than before?

I had not thought of this until just now. In my late twenties I took a trip to Africa and had the opportunity to see a witch doctor, in his little teepee sitting on a loin cloth with his granddaughter interpreting. I noticed a half-full bottle of what may have been wine next to him but it could have been anything. His eyes gazed through me. He took my hands, touched and pushed slightly on my wrists and my forehead. He had a stone bowl with a stone dowel that he ground together for several minutes. He closed his eyes then began speaking. His granddaughter shared with me that I would be old but will have many joint and back pains and will have some suffering from this.

(There were other things, but this is relevant since I was referred to you by a friend when I was in horrid pain and could not even turn over in bed at the age of thirty. I was very impressed walking into your clinic in Newport Beach and saw large framed pictures of every famous sports personality I could imagine. Football, tennis, skiing, Olympic gold medal winners, ballerinas, body builders including Arnold, gold medal winners in swimming, soccer, rugby, and so on. I was amazed. I had no idea how you did what you did. After one treatment of injections in my bone on bone lower discs, you said, "Do these little exercises and give it six months." I was completely cured in three months and the follow up x-ray showed the new cartilage and bone growth. No more pain and I was thrilled. You were and are my hero.)

Face to face with the witch doctor, I'd had quite a few injuries and emergency events, all having to do with shoulder, hips, pelvis, and back. (I fell off the back of a moving motorcycle, flew off a swing and flew through the air, while carrying a big box to my car I tripped over a speed bump and broke a leg and hip.)

Without my being able to follow Dr. Ongley wherever he had his clinic, I would be permanently in a wheelchair or seriously addicted to painkillers and a drug junkie by now. I experienced firsthand what this amazingly kind and loving man has done for me, and his hundreds and thousands of patients all over the world. It is forty-two years after my first visit and he is still helping me stay in shape and pain free.

Dr. Ongley

I am only doing what I came here to do, but thank you. Getting back to what we are doing here—I knew an old friend at the Optimum Health Institute in San Diego, California and he was afflicted with cancer in the pancreas. I had known him as an

Olympian athlete and in his competitive days. Absolutely nothing would stop him from doing his training to exhaustion. He was the most selfish person in the world from my point of view. "No matter what happens, I must do this," he would tell me. Most great athletes have to have the drive, as I well know from my days of mastering the art of swimming and rugby internationally. Everything else is secondary, except for me—medicine was number one.

I remember talking to him at the clinic in San Diego. I was saying goodbye and he was going off to have his evening meal and he turned around to me. He said, "This time next year I will be dead." I nearly stopped in my tracks and I said, "Goodbye, Gordon." He turned and looked me right in the eye and said goodbye.

Now, our relationship had always been, no matter where we met around the world I said, "Goodbye, Gordon." He would catch a plane or whatever he had to do and I would do the same thing. That was his way. This time it was his way of telling me he wasn't going off to catch a plane. He was going to die.

Sieglinde
Did he die?

Dr. Ongley
Oh yes, and within the year. And yet on the same day at the Optimum Health Institute halfway through our afternoon as usual he was always wearing a track suit, put on his jogging shoes and went off and jogged several miles. Yet, whatever it was within him in spite of his continuing his training and his jogging, he wanted to die.

. . .

Sieglinde

He believed he would die.

Dr. Ongley

He either believed, knew, or talked himself into it. We know that to overcome cancer of the pancreas, which he had, is a killer. But my impression of this very good friend was that he had simply decided and that was very sad.

I had persuaded him to leave England just at the height of his fame after winning silver medals at the Melbourne Olympics and migrate to New Zealand and we became close friends. He enjoyed himself there thoroughly. But on this particular occasion when I met him in San Diego, he had telephoned me at the office right out of the blue as usual. "Here I am; what are you doing." He had searched the world looking for a place that might help him and he found the Optimum Health center. The problem is you cannot help someone who has made up his mind to die. He was returning to England, and he never left.

Sieglinde

This is very sad. It feels to me that you gave him the sweetness of life through your friendship. This is the emotion of the pancreas and his medals may not have given him enough of the true sweetness of life. Diabetics also love to eat too much sugar to fill the void for missing the sweet God-given nectar of life.

. . .

What is the point of a doctor telling a patient about the severity of the disease?

Dr. Ongley

A doctor's job should be to seek the truth. If doctors would seek the truth as humanely as possible, of course side by side, with their patients, we should not have so much skull duggers in the healing arts that we have.

Sieglinde

What is skull dugger?

Dr. Ongley

I was reading a newspaper article that talked about back pain and how it afflicted eighty percent of the population and how it is a $60 billion industry in the United States. Just reading the comment of the reporter who interviewed the various patients and doctors gave me the impression that the article mentioned at least twenty different ways of taking care of the average back pain. The different approaches were so contrary—I think I mentioned to you previously that one patient will be saying that you have to bend forward all the time to get rid of your back pain; the next person says, bend backwards all the time and let's see if that gets rid of your back pain. If that doesn't work, lie on the floor and push your pelvis up, do pelvic tilts. No one of those prospects will use the test of his therapy. Does it actually cure back pain—can that person return to his former advocation, pain free? If they were to face the truth and use that as a test, if everyone used the same test then we could evaluate the different therapies correctly.

. . .

Sieglinde

I'm surprised. Everything is regulated—why is it so difficult to regulate orthopedic work when the Ongley method is so simple?

Dr. Ongley

Again, you have choice if you are sane or insane.

Sieglinde

Are the Chinese better healers?

Dr. Ongley

Do they live any longer and do they have any less health problems than anyone else? Again, this is another one of those things coming from Hijanjanakopan. Someone hears a radio program and says, "I've gotta have that mushroom or that drink." If it's mystical and difficult to get ahold of, people always want more and they demand it. This is the human way. This is why you have so many court battles about people who believe that if you put blood into their veins to save a baby's life it's hell or damnation, so you elect to let the baby die.

Many years ago I was one of the first people to go around shouting, "Yes we do have the right to die as much as we have the right to live." This has now become sort of a watchword today: "Yes, we have the right to die." At that point in time when you make that decision are you sane? Health professionals have said this right to die is marvelous if it's made by a sane person at the time. All you have to do is get a sixteen-year-old girl who's been dumped by her boyfriend and she wants to die. But does she have the right to do that? Yes, she has the right, but was she sane at the time? Of course not. As soon as she finds another boyfriend, now she wants to live. This is a big problem. I will not shout out saying the FDA and the AMA is utterly worthless because it is not. There just happens to be a lot of skull duggery going on in medicine and in every other facet of human existence. You need these institutions, you need medical school, or else you have the rule where a young person becomes an apprentice to a doctor like a plumber and he leads by apprenticeship.

Sieglinde

So are you back to the simplistic approach? "Mother knows best" does not apply here. Only you know what's best for you and your body.

Dr. Ongley

That is the point.

Sieglinde

How do we become better doctors for ourselves?

Dr. Ongley

We must learn the language of medicine and our body. The reason for that is if you go to the doctor and you have a pain running down your leg, he looks at you and he strokes his beard and seems to understand that pain going down the leg immediately translates the pain into the language of medicine and says, "You have sciatica." Now you go say, "I have sciatica." You go home and tell everyone, "I have sciatica." If you know the language of medi-cine and understand it, you will start to see the good and the bad points that are in medicine in general and you can take responsibility for your own actions.

Another one of my complaints is that we all have to live by the law. When I went to school I was taught the subjects of medicine, foreign languages, et cetera, but no one taught me the law. No one knows all of the laws. In the same way why don't we, in school, learn more about our bodies? In this modern age it would be a great advantage through our personal computers if we hook into a central computer where we put in our symptoms and the computer tells us how to take care of the simple diseases in life. If this computer was in a drugstore the patients come in, punch in the symptoms, and they get the medicine dictated to them. Now you have freed up doctors of ninety percent of their mundane chores. They can spend their time doing the very serious aspects of medicine. I don't have a crystal ball but I see this happening—and I would love it to happen.

Sieglinde

This sounds good. I must, however, share a personal experience. A few years ago I was referred to a doctor and she came into the little exam room with her iPad. She asked me a few questions and busily input them into her laptop; the whole time she never looked at me. Then out came a group of medications she will prescribe to me and left. I thought there would be more so I waited. Suddenly another patient was put in the room and I left without a word. This is not what you are talking about, is it?

Dr. Ongley

No it is not. I will make what I said more clear. At this time there are computerized gloves so that the surgeon in the middle of

Russia someplace can put on his gloves, and through his computer he can put his hand over the patient and tell exactly what to do. This is happening so all we need now is for all of the world's specialists to be hooked up to the central computer so the public can go in, get immediate feedback with, let's say a tiny green light and the pharmacist can prescribe. If there is a red light it says you must be seen. So and so. This becomes a sorting station, freeing up the family practitioner.

Now you could get clever and lie to the computer, but how is that different from people who lie to their doctors for a certain prescription, or to get a certificate to go back to work or to say, "I need disability income from the state." Once the patient has suckered the doctor into giving him a form or treatment, now the patient is controlling the doctor. The patient can make up his mind as to how he wants the treatment to work. If you are in the field of manipulation and if you, the doctor, are tricked by the patient into manipulating him who has nothing wrong, he can say, "Well it was better but now it's worse." If the doctor says, "I cannot see any indication for manipulation," now the doctor is in control and he will not manipulate.

Sieglinde

How large a percentage of people go to a doctor if there is nothing wrong? People have quite an investment in being sick. Children learn early to get attention when sick. They are mothered and pampered and get attention. The benefits of ill health are learned conditioned responses early in life.

Dr. Ongley

It was Winston Churchill who said, "Half of the work was done by people not feeling well." Now if we ever get the other half of the work done by the people in the world who say, "I'm sick" and stay home, this would be interesting, would it not?

Sieglinde

How does pain protect?

Dr. Ongley

If the child puts the finger on the hot plate, he feels pain and pulls it away. You can sit in front of an electric heater and feel the burn, the pain.

Sieglinde

Why do some people enjoy pain? What happens to these people?

Dr. Ongley

These people are insane. Or they are wrapped up in a popular trend, coming along where the people are going this way and either it works and finds a new path or it stops. Some religious cults, where we are indoctrinated about pain being punishment, they have to suffer. That's where the word *pain* brought in punishment or penalty.

There has to be eventual progress for them. Unfortunately anybody who deviates just a little from the mainstream to try to make progress, they are ostracized. So the inevitable, very slow mainstream approach must now become mainstream. It will continue at a slower rate from the person who whips out here to find a new pathway. Why must they be so hard on the renegades that try to find a new and easier pathway? Why must mainstream medicine be so hard on the innovative provided they are not out there harming? Provided they are not harming, why should they not try to create new pathways? If you read the history of heart transplants and cardiac surgery in general you will find that the pioneers were killing people right and left. A British surgeon managed to kill so many patients that he said, "I throw in the towel, it is my job to save people, not kill them."

In mainstream medicine you've asked me to do this work and I can't face it anymore. They said, "Wait a minute, you have so much experience killing people; we want you to continue." They rallied around him and got him back working and he began to solve the problems and he began to save lives. So there is an example where mainstream medicine did not ostracize the innovator.

We haven't mentioned Sam Weiss; he was working in the field of obstetrics and in his town there was a building in which he delivered babies. While waiting for the mother to come to term, the doctors would go down and do post-mortems. Then someone called Dr. Weiss and said, "She is about to give birth" and he would wipe his hands on his apron and of course infect the patient and many died. So he went to the medical profession and he wasted little time watching the girls, the midwives. The girls seemed to always be washing their hands, keeping everything very clean. Of course, these were the days before Pasteur. The girls didn't have the insignia of the butcher, they didn't wear these aprons.

He maintained to the medical profession that they should wash their hands and he ended up in an insane institution because he was talking about things that have to be up in the air. Things no one can see. If you can't see something it doesn't exist—"The man is ridiculous." This is typical of the history of medicine.

Sieglinde

Wouldn't it be great if we could look into a crystal ball and see all of the things not yet discovered or utilized? There must be unimaginable things that other cultures in other parts of our galaxy take as common.

Dr. Ongley

Sure it would. Everyone dealing with the unknown, something outside of their medical religion, or what others don't understand is persecuted.

Anyone who is an innovator, working in the field of medicine that is unseen and unknown, is persecuted by peers and the medical society. They have one set of rules and yet another for the rest of the people.

Anybody who is an innovator and is making progress should be supported, not chopped off. If you look at Hageman, the Father of Homeopathy, when the plague was rushing through Europe he was the one person who was able to have something of a reasonable success rate with the plague. But his prescription, being so cheap, that the pharmacists all banned together and put up the money to get Hageman out of Germany. He lived and died in France. If you read the history of medicine you will see how the so-called establishment in medicine, the ivory tower, *is what's wrong in medicine*.

. . .

Sieglinde

Beside the power and money, why are they so threatened by innovators? They supposedly all share the same oath, to heal.

Dr. Ongley

Now we are back to ego.

Sieglinde

What is keeping more doctors from using your method for curing pain permanently?

Dr. Ongley

Lack of knowledge. Everyone wants a better method to treat their patients. All physicians love the patient lording over them when the pain is gone. We humans seem to like that. I have been teaching people all over the world, but have no idea how many people are using it. Compared to forty years ago, much progress has been made in physicians attempting to using the method I have developed all around the world.

Sieglinde

What do you mean attempting?

Dr. Ongley

It is like playing a piano. I don't watch them treat patients, I don't know how skillful they are. The same applies to me. The other fellow doesn't know how skillful I am. Again, the only test there is, is the result. If people are getting a good result then they are doing an adequate job. They might be able to do a better job or they might be worse. If people are getting well then the physician is doing his job.

Sieglinde

You know your clients get well and are free of pain.

Dr. Ongley

The discussion is not about me. The discussion is about methods.

Sieglinde

You have such a problem being honored and recognized.

Dr. Ongley

What do you mean, it's not a question of being recognized. Nothing is new under the sun—we all agree on that. What is recognition, who wants it? What is it? Who needs so-called human recognition? We decided a long time ago, either you are a helper or not a helper. You don't want recognition when you help someone. Why put a different set of rules on me?

Sieglinde

I get frustrated with your humbleness. I know how great you are and I would love for everyone to know about you and to have the experience of being healed by you. Also to have every patient demanding your treatment.

Dr. Ongley

That's your opinion. Just as many people wouldn't say that.

Sieglinde

Not patients, maybe other people, but they are the ones we are talking about.

Dr. Ongley

Now you are qualifying people. We care about all people. There is nothing good or bad. Only thinking makes it so. Provided that professionals are out there helping patients, whether they are using the same techniques or the same type of treatment than I am using, doesn't matter as long as they are getting results and patients are getting well.

Sieglinde

In orthopedic medicine, are people becoming pain free?

Dr. Ongley

But they are, in orthopedic medicine, not orthopedic surgery.

Sieglinde

It seems that hip and knee replacements have grown by leaps and bounds in the last forty years and are often quite successful.

Dr. Ongley

No it is not. It is helping people. I am simply saying that if surgeons had more knowledge and more treatments available, maybe some of the surgeries could be prevented. It all comes down to knowledge. If you go to mechanic A and your carburetor is not good, he will simply replace it. Mechanic B, it takes longer in time but he will go right through the carburetor and clean it up, renew this and that.

Sieglinde

But there is more money in a new carburetor and the installation.

Dr. Ongley

Yes. You give me the alternative. Put a new carburetor on while you wait and go *vroom*. So the question is it better to put in a new one—that is your decision. The same dilemma is found in medicine. For people who have the money, they want a new one slapped in.

Sieglinde

So we keep going around the same bush. There really is no answer to it, is there?

Dr. Ongley

You got it. We have pointed out that the FDA is necessary but it can be bought. Established medicine is necessary. It is necessary today because in other days you didn't have telephones, fax machines, or TV or the internet, which replaces libraries et cetera, computers, iPhones, and tablets. In those days nobody knew what the hell you were doing anyhow. So as long as you were the witch doctor in the little village and hemmed in by mountains, no one criticized you. He did his best, which isn't a bad set of rules. He did his best. My complaint is too many people are not doing their best.

So now he throws in big words like *holistic medical care*, *alternative medicine*, the *right* of the human being. Now with the advent of the world getting smaller and smaller, we are finding out that these people are not doing their best.

Sieglinde

Was this not the seed for people taking more responsibility for their health through knowledge?

Dr. Ongley

That is the ultimate.

Sieglinde

Who will teach people to be their own physician?

Dr. Ongley

Was it really necessary for all of us to be doing trigonometry and calculus? Today kids are doing it with calculators or they Google it. We have gone too far. Maybe we need another world war to make things speed up, to force the change needed in our educational system.

Sieglinde

Maybe there will be another disaster that will speed things up. Possibly through mother nature or the cosmos around us.

Dr. Ongley

Is this that much different than war? It will kill people. In order to save yourself in whatever field to beat the enemy off, even mother nature. This is called rapid progression.

Sieglinde

Will this human notion of having a bigger club than the next person ever stop?

Dr. Ongley

How can it ever stop? There is only X amount of what the individual human wants. It is limited and as you get more and more humans wanting, whether it is gold or coal or whatever, there won't be enough. So when you're ill and starving then Jack will have to kill John to get his food. This does not necessarily refer to food; it can be gold, the fuel, his woman, whatever.

Sieglinde

So you are saying greed is a part of human nature. I hope that as we advance in our consciousness we can override these needs for greed, blame, shame, jealousy.

Dr. Ongley

Sure it is. Let me ask you this: Were you born greedy? I don't think so. The answer to all of this is like everything. Quite simple. Humans must stop the greed. You also can't keep on having the population explode when there might not be enough for every single person everywhere on this planet.

Sieglinde

But there is enough to go around.

. . .

Dr. Ongley

Do you really think the man with the tummy full is going to go to Somalia to see the man who is starving? Every political leader that I have knowledge of, he realizes there is not enough gold to pay the army or whatever it is that supports him. He realizes this and says, "Oh, I don't have enough gold. If I give up all of my gold to the soldiers, there is not enough left for me." So he says, "I will pretend that there is more gold. Now how can I pretend that there is more gold than there is? I'll give you all markers or money that represents gold."

Sieglinde

We are back to the illusion of it all.

Dr. Ongley

Yes, and it is also an illusion that there is enough of anything to go around for too long. When a glimpse of the illusion rises to the surface, the political leader is out.

The man in Texas demands five thousand acres for himself. You tell that to a man in Japan where space is at a premium. Now because the world is small, the Japanese man will come running to Texas saying, "I don't need all of that space, we need it." The Texan says, "No, you just run back to where you come from. I need my five thousand acres." Then he says, "Well if you won't give it up, we will take it." "Oh no you're not." He pulls out his .44 and they pull out their big swords and they go to battle.

. . .

That's how it is. Why have the Mormons become so unpopular in the days of the old Wild West? The men had seven wives, they come to a town dragging their carts with seven women behind them, a town of only men.

The question we are playing is what happens to humans when one has and the other has not. The fellow who has not will find any number of reasons to take from the one who has. Another example might be if you have fifteen cars. You can't look after them all, you have to lock them up in a big shed. You need a guard to watch them. People will come along and will try to steal them. They will want to take them from you.

Sieglinde

Will people revert back to a simple respectful life? A life where there is honor and respect for all things.

Dr. Ongley

Not if you have the numbers we have on the planet today.

Sieglinde

So population numbers must be decreased.

Dr. Ongley

That's the way I see it.

Sieglinde

There has been much said by the powers to be on this planet about depopulation.

Dr. Ongley

Yes, and who will select who will live and who will die?

Sieglinde

Hopefully someone bigger than you or I but presently the powers controlling us all have no emotional component making them capable of choosing wisely and humanely.

Dr. Ongley

I sure wouldn't want the responsibility or the knowledge. Obviously it is about supply and demand. If the supply cannot keep up with the demand, you have a problem. This is the bottom line, regardless of the reason.

Sieglinde

If the me-me attitude stopped and people were happy and life is enjoyed and embraced just as it is now, what would change?

Dr. Ongley

Progress today is a century ahead of what we are shown and space travel and living on other planets is close by, so is cloning and making humans into drones possibly controlled by robots. There are many possibilities in the works.

· · ·

Getting back to now. If you go to a person who bases his life on worldly possessions, he says you're nuts. "I want the big house, fancy cars, jewels, my big bank account offshore and my ten wives," whatever. They all think this is absolutely essential for them. So now you need your own security guards which become your personal army. The fellow next door is thirty-two, he sees you at sixty and you have this big army, you've got everything including your own island. "I want a piece of that action," so he comes along and starts a war with you. It gives you a heart attack and you die. He takes over.

Sieglinde

What is the point of this madness everywhere?

Dr. Ongley

To me there is no point. Humans are only relatively happy while they are getting it. You either cut yourself adrift from this so-called madness and rub shoulders with it only when necessary, but then you have reduced the number of problems that you as an individual have. We have pointed out the futility of it all once you're into it, it goes on and on and on. There is no win. You must jump out. It is impossible to stay out in its entirety, then take it in very small doses.

Sieglinde

With all of the corruption in the world throughout time, why does it continue?

Dr. Ongley

It is a game. Do you really think they wanted to eliminate Saddam Hussein they couldn't. This is why North Koreans say, "You put down your nuclear arms and we won't strive to get one." We say that's wrong. "We can have it but you can't." This is part of the game here if you want to play. You have a choice, however, to be it in the game or not.

Sieglinde

What if the population does not choose the game? I have always hoped everyone would stand up and say, "Enough already." When I know that you know what I am thinking, the jig is up and there is no place to hide the lie.

Dr. Ongley

Most governments would topple. If you said, "Okay, we want to analyze the taxation. We won't pay the tax."

The government says, "Wait a minute, who is going to pay my wages? Who is going to pay for my girlfriend?" We pointed out previously the power is within the individual. He has the power to vote, he can do it. But they are so dammed stupid and so dammed smug that they won't exercise it. They actually believe that the examination of the Clinton's guilt is going on. They are at the bottom of the list of innocent and the top of the list of the guilty. If they are to make it they will whitewash, acid erase computers and burn evidence and do away with persons who may tell anything that may look bad for them.

Sieglinde

I don't believe it's possible to be a politician in this country or anywhere else and not be dirty.

.   .   .

Dr. Ongley

It is impossible.

Sieglinde

Why do people think they are superior and special when they only tell you what you want to hear so they stay in office for life?

Dr. Ongley

Because there is something so stupid in humans that the person in power isn't just a human like the rest of us. He brushes his teeth like the rest of us. He is the same. We are making him different in our minds. When the Queen of England walks in, why should we bow down? Think about it. What is so different about her?

In my youth, my family belonged to the many private clubs in England. I swam in the royal swimming pool and I called her Lizzy and her sister, Maggie, would jump in the pool with me. We had great fun as I went on to be an internationally known swimmer. We must begin to face the truth about all things. If you are steeped in British tradition and you analyze those people who are being knighted or honored, they are not different than anyone else.

Sieglinde

Why do we need heroes?

Dr. Ongley

It is not hero worship, it is envy. This reminds me of the planet of the apes. When Charlton Heston is going up the hill from the crashed spaceship, he turns around and says, "There has to be something better." This is why I'm on a mission. There has to be something better.

Sieglinde

Maybe this is it. How do we get out of our heads and into our hearts and into a state of neutrality?

Dr. Ongley

Get rid of the mythology. Mythology is that when the little girl is born you call her my princess and she will find a prince charming and they will live happily ever after. These are myths. Anatomically there are boys and there are girls. Let's start there. That's it. Let's get rid of the mythology that you have to have a union.

You must have the rights of the individuals, you cannot do what China has done where they kill off the female children because they all want a boy. Since they can only have one child, the male is preferred and upheld as the warrior. This is wrong. People have the right to overpopulate and they have the right to starve. But don't tell me about my unborn baby. You'll go through that one until the cows come home. I have a right.

Did you hear about the woman who got kicked out of a shopping mall because she was breastfeeding her baby in public? So everyone was arguing about it. One guy stood up and said, "You should be modest. Go to the bathroom and feed the baby." She thought she was clever and said, "Would you like to have your breakfast in the bathroom?" People clapped. Someone else said, "Why not build a room for nursing mothers." It might be okay for the woman to say, "We all know we have breasts and we feed babies with breasts but to some this is offensive, so I understand that." The woman said, "Well I don't care" and the other person said, "Well I do care. So don't ram her ideas down his throat or vice versa." That is very hard to do, isn't it?

In my lifetime the mere thought of how woman got a baby was taboo, you simply did not did not talk about it. Maybe they were found under a mulberry bush—you see, this was a great mystery in the past. There are still people out there who are not liberated in this world. They are still wearing veils up to their eyes. They don't show that a girl has an ankle. Now you go to one of those countries and you decide to breastfeed your baby in public. So let's have consideration for others.

So they took a whole bunch of mothers to the shopping mall breastfeeding all of their babies. A sit-in. Women want to show you "I have a baby and not only that, it is the best baby in the world. My baby will have everything in the world, you are going to pay for it, but mine will have everything."

Sieglinde

This comes from women thinking they own the baby, that the child belongs to them forever.

Dr. Ongley

You and I understand that the mother is simply the vehicle. The mother will not believe this. Now the mother says, "My child needs this gold and your child doesn't." Then she will bash your head in to get it.

. . .

Sieglinde

Everything seems to be a mystery when we don't understand.

Dr. Ongley

If you will adopt the philosophies that we have been hinting at, to realize there's no big mystery, no big secret.

When it comes down to the mystery, it is not just the philosophy of life. You can take something small like the mystique of a woman. That is no big mystery, is it now? You sit there and laugh. It is all nonsense. It is all in our head. Stop worshiping false gods, stop running after and stop worshiping the false gods.

Sieglinde

Why do we need to own and claim everything as our own?

Dr. Ongley

You have got to be joking. That is the easiest one in the world. If the government owns people—and they do—and forces them to work, and if the government takes the fruits of their labors, they are very rich. That is how it is. You go back to work, don't smell the roses. Oh no. "You produce and I will get it for you. I will take the produce or I will let you sell it and take your money or most of it." Whether you like it or not, you're working for the government.

You must come to the realization of what it's all about. The truth, the acceptance, and do your best within yourself. Do what you want to do when you feel like doing it, provided you are harming no one.

Only thinking makes it so. Beware of your thoughts—always come from love, never fear.

Sieglinde

It seems the world is only a projection. Time is one moment and we seem to be banished into ignorance in this dimension. Thank you so much for your insight, Dr. Ongley.

Chapter Three

ARTICLES BY DR. ONGLEY

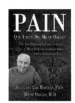

Chapter Four

ORTHOPAEDIC MEDICINE

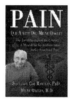

INSTITUTE OF ORTHOPAEDIC MEDICINE

Musculo-Skeletal Injection Therapy

The technique of injecting specific solutions into body tissues for reparative purposes has been used by physicians for more than 150 years. Varicose veins, hernias, and hemorrhoids were treated by this method in the late 1930's in the United States.

The results of these early injections clearly indicated that growth of new tissue did occur following administration. Various commercial preparations of solutions were available to physicians but none proved to be entirely satisfactory in all medical aspects.

Milne Ongley, a New Zealand physician, prepared laboratory variations of a number of proliferant preparations to develop a safe and effective solution for use on his patients. After controlled laboratory trials and clinical evaluations of the resultant healing and strengthening of the musculo-skeletal tissue, he succeeded in formulating a solution that met the medical criteria of safety, effectively, and patient tolerance. He also perfected a specialized injection technique that is far superior to the earlier methods of injection, and one that accelerated the healing and strengthening effects of the solution. This solution is medically well accepted, used by physicians, and referred to in medical literature as Ongley's Solution; his injection technique is labeled Ongley's Technique. Upon request, Ongley taught his proven technique to interested physicians in New Zealand, South Africa, Great Britain, the United States and other countries.

Since the introduction of Ongley's Solution to the practice of orthopaedic medicine, hundreds of thousands of these injections have been given by physicians throughout the world into injured joints of the neck, back, shoulder, hip, knee, ankle, wrist, and into other smaller joints with no recorded serious side effects and with highly successful therapeutic results. This beneficial injectable solution has a well-established record of medical safety and reliability.

The injection therapy is designed to aid tissue repair and to restore stability to the affected joint. Ongley designed a series of specialized exercises which are an essential part of the treatment and rehabilitation and aid in the more rapid tissue growth and in the subsequent healing and restoration of movement to the affected joints.

Ongley's Solution is composed of ingredients that are standard to the practice of medicine. Before being injected, these ingredients are diluted with an equal amount of local anesthetic solution. The injection initially causes an inflammatory reaction that facilitates the migration of specialized fibroblast cells to the injected area. The fibroblasts then produce new collagen in the affected portion of the body and stimulate the subsequent growth of new collagen tissue. The collagen tissue cell growth strengthens the basic structure of the injured portion of the body.

A double-blind study that presented further confirmation of the efficacy and reliability of Ongley's Solution and injection technique was completed in Santa Barbara, California. The study provided statistically significant information that indicated physical improvement in the overwhelming majority of patients treated for chronic low-back pain. The results of the study were published in the

LANCET, a British medical journal, in July 1987. This publication brings professional and public recognition to the long-known positive effects of correctly administered and completed musculoskeletal injection therapy using Ongley's Solution and Ongley's Technique.

For maximum healing and for joint mobility it is essential to exercise as directed and prescribed following each injection. The new tissue formation will grow and strengthen, and with the advice and consent of the treating physician one is able to enjoy walking, cycling, swimming or favorite sports. The body is able to respond to and benefit from a unique and highly specialized method of treatment as practiced by physicians skilled in this technique.

This explanation of musculoskeletal injection therapy is presented as a general overview. If you have specific questions about treatment, your physician will gladly provide detailed answers.

Protected by Copyright Act of 1958.

INSTITUTE OF ORTHOPAEDIC MEDICINE

Chapter Five

BACK SHOT

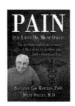

BACK SHOT

Dr. Milne Ongley's cure for backache

By Tom Deters, DC.

For this segment in our back pain series, I traveled to the Institute of Orthopaedic Medicine in Newport Beach, California, to report on a revolutionary new procedure for the treatment of chronic low back pain called "Researched and developed by Milne Ongley, this method uses the injection of a special solution that has been shown to strengthen weak ligaments and restore lower back stability.

By Tom Deters, DC. Managing Publisher

As I scanned the office walls, my eyes focused on two plaques. One was an award for an "Outstanding contribution to Orthopaedic medicine" and the other was for "Outstanding service and professionalism."

Prestigious awards indeed, presented to a man for many years of distinguished achievement.

I remembered my time at school. I was fascinated by the research of Kirkaldy-Willis, Haldeman and Fienstein. All these scientists devoted their research to low back pain and the precise *mechanism* for spinal dysfunction. They were pioneers in my field. I was about to meet another. Joe Weider had sent me to interview the British physician Milne Ongley at this Newport Beach office. Dr. Ongley developed Ongley's technique, which *was* the hot topic at the American Back Society convention in San Francisco this past year. Turns out that Joe and Ongley were old friends (is there anyone in the health and fitness field who isn't a friend of Joe's?) from the time Joe supplied Ongley's Olympic athletes with protein powders in England. Free of charge, as Ongley pointed out. Ongley was training and treating some of the world finest track and field athletes at the time, meanwhile picking the Master Blaster's brain for the latest in training information. He was also making major breakthroughs in the field of orthopaedics. That was 30 years ago!

It has always amused me that scientists in laboratories often receive the credit for explaining things that others have felt to be true for years. I don't mean to belittle research discoveries, but science can only work with the elements that the real world provides. A "white coat stamp of approval" often comes after the fact. More than a ball a century ago bodybuilders were talking about the health benefits they received from lifting weights, but it is only accepted as truth today because scientists are now publishing articles on the "Physiological Benefits of Isolcinetic Resistance Therapy" (weight training).

Ongley also had to wait until science caught up. It wasn't until July 1987, when The Lancet (an elite British medical journal) published the results of a double-blind study on Ongley's solution and chronic low back pain that gave Ongley's solution and Ongley's technique the recognition it so justly deserved.

The study provided statistically significant *data that showed improvement in the vast majority* of patients treated for chronic low back pain with a series of injections with a special solution designed to tighten ligaments and stabilize joints. (A ligament is a thick band of connective tissue that connects two bones together in the area of a joint, as opposed to a tendon which attaches a muscle to a bone). The technique of injecting specific solutions into body tissues for reparative purposes has been used by physicians for more than ISO years. Varicose veins, hernias and hemorrhoids have been treated by this method since the 1930s in the United States. However, none of these solutions was able to stimulate tire growth of new tissue.

Ongley extensively researched the conceit of proliferant therapy. He was interested in developing a solution that he could inject into ligaments that would make them stronger and thicker, thereby offering more stability to the joints they summated. He wanted this thickening to result from the development of additional ligamentous tissue- not scar tissue, which is not as strong or as durable as the regular tissue. If ligaments that had been torn, stretched ©r otherwise injured were tightened, the patient would be able to resume activity that previously would have continued to damage the joints, leading to arthritis.

After years of laboratory trials and clinical testing Ongley developed a solution and an injection technique that accelerated healing, strengthened ligaments and was safe. He began using this formula in 1956. Since that time, hundreds of thousands of these injections have been given by physicians throughout the world in the treatment of injuries of the neck, back, shoulder, hip, knee, ankle and wrist with no recorded serious side effects and excellent results. Ongley has taught his technique to other doctors in New Zealand, South Africa, Great Britain and the United States.

ONGLEY BEATS A BAD BACK

Low back pain is estimated to affect 80% of the United States population. Treatment includes exercise, massage, acupuncture, physiotherapy, chiropractic, drugs and surgery. Chronic or recurring low back pain is often the most difficult to treat successfully because it can have so many causes. Whale chiropractic treatment is often successful, depending on the individual's condition, *relief* from many forms of treatment is only temporary. Years of cumulative trauma from injury, improper lifting technique or abuse can stress or loosen the spinal ligaments, creating instability and excessive wear and tear on the spinal joints disks. Ongley believes that by identifying the area of instability. Mobilizing the involved joints to ensure proper function and then strengthening or "tightening" the ligaments, he can eventually solve the problem. Ongley's technique *has* been proven successful in treating chronic low back pain.

I spent a day with Ongley and his partner, Dr. Louis Schlom, observing this technique for low back treatment from start to finish. Ongley begins by reviewing the patient's medical history. He then checks X-rays and gives the patient an extensive physical orthopedic and neurological exam, paying particular attention to posture and biomechanies. Ongley then tells the patient what he has found out and what he plans *to* do about it.

Typically for low back pain, Ongley will manipulate the area to make sum the joint is moving correctly and then he will administer the first of eight weekly injections of Ongley's solution. He has the patient perform special exercises immediately after each treatment to maintain flexibility and resume the full range of motion to the joint Mote often than not, Ongley reports, this eight-week program does the trick, but occasionally a person may require an additional injection or two to get the desired results.

This treatment regimen is recognized as being safe by the medical community and the chance of serious side effects is remote. After therapy, patients may experience some discomfort or stiffness, or may have some bruising at the point of injection.

NEW HOPE FOR THE FUTURE

Ongley's technique has provided results to patients who have tried everything under the sun for back problems. This procedure has been successfully applied to strengthen ligaments in many other joints as well.

Two of the most commonly injured joints are the shoulder and the knee. Both of these joints rely heavily on the surrounding muscles as well as ligaments for their support and as such have *been* treated effectively with Ongley's technique. For many years the common treatment for damaged ligaments of the knee has been major reconstructive surgery where a portion of a tendon was grafted onto the injured area, or the ligament was replaced with synthetic material.

This type of surgery has been successful, but requires an extensive rehabilitation program. Ongley reports that he has had good results with treating knees having severely damaged ligaments. He has had similar successes in treating unstable joints of the hip, shoulder, wrist, neck and ankle.

In years to come we may be able to control arthritis and orthopaedic problems with a short series of injections and a solid course of exercise. After all, there's always hope with guys like Milne Ongley around, so anything is possible.

Chapter Six

LANCET ARTICLE

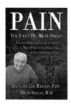

Reprinted from THE LANCET, July 18, 1987. pp. 143–146.

A NEW APPROACH TO THE TREATMENT OF CHRONIC LOW BACK PAIN

MILNE J. ONGLEY, ROBERT G. KLEIN, THOMAS A. DORMAN, BJORN C. EEK, LAWRENCE J. HUBERT

Department of Rheumatology, Sansum Medical Clinic, and the Sansum Medical Research Foundation, Santa Barbara, California 93102, USA

Summary 81 patients with chronic low back pain (average duration 10 years) were randomised to two treatment groups. Forty received an empirically devised regimen of forceful spinal manipulation and injections of adextrose-glycerine-phenol ("proliferant") solution into soft-tissue structures, as part of a programme to decrease pain and disability. The other 41 patients received parallel treatment in which the main differences were less extensive initial local anaesthesia and manipulation, and substitution of saline for proliferant. Neither patients nor assessors knew which treatment had been given. When assessed by disability scores the experimental group had greater improvement than the control group at one ($p < 0.001$), three ($p < 0.004$), and six ($p < 0.001$) months from the end of treatment; at six months an improvement of more than 50% was recorded in 35 of the experimental group versus 16 of the control group and the numbers free from disability were 15 and 4, respectively (p < 0·003). Visual analogue pain scores and pain diagrams likewise showed significant advantages for the experimental regimen.

INTRODUCTION

Over thirty years ago, one of us (M. J. O.) tried the effect of repeated epidural injections of local anaesthetic agents in patients with low back pain, on the supposition that most such pain was secondary to irritation of the Jura or nerve roots. This treatment was rarely successful. Other pain-sensitive soft-tissue structures were then systematically evaluated by local anaesthesia, and it emerged that the ligaments and soft tissues of the low back were of primary import. At about the same time, Hackett' was injecting ligaments with various chemical agents in the hope of causing fibroblast hyperplasia and thus increasing their strength. When he claimed a cure rate of 82% in 1600 patients with low back pain, other physicians took up the treatment, but progress in this area was retarded by reports of 3 cases of paralysis and 2 deaths after inadvertent injection of material (psyllium seed oil and zinc sulphate) into the subarachnoid space.[6-8.] On the theory that all sclerosants work in same way, by causing an inflammatory response and thus fibroblast proliferation leading to new collagen production, M. J. chose to use dextrose-glycerine-phenol solution, originally developed for treatment of varicose veins; it has a good safety record and causes little pain.

A treatment system was developed empirically, the main of which were injection of dilute lignocaine to interrupt the pain reflex arc, a single forceful manipulation to ensure full range of movement, injection of "proliferant" solution into specific fascial and ligamentous sites, "disinflammation" of any accompanying glutealirritati with a single injection of corticosteroid, and repeated flexion exercises.

. . .

We have assessed this regimen in a double-blind trial. Because of the complexity of the regimen we departed from the traditional double-blind protocol in which only a single variable is s died. Instead we tested the entire system against a control system modified to include some but not all features of the full treatment programme.

PATIENTS AND METHODS

Patient Selection

Solicitations were mailed to 10 000 previously registered patients of the Sansum Medical Clinic (a multispecialty group), selected randomly and without regard to previous complaints of back pain.

This was a computer-generated list based on zip codes. Patients were informed of the nature of the study and were invited to apply to participate if they had back pain of more than one year in duration that had not responded to previous conservative (non-surgical) treatment. Two hundred twenty-eight applications were returned. Patients were not interviewed if they were less than 21 or more than 70 years old, if they were pregnant or contemplating pregnancy, if they had litigation pending if they had an unsettled worker's compensation **claim, or if they were on disability pay. Other reasons for rejection before interview; were body weight more than 25% over ideal** (making injections technically more difficult), insulin-dependent diabetes, coronary artery disease, and debilitating **medical** conditions. Patients were arbitrarily excluded if they had fewer than 4 positive responses on the disability pain questionnaire (see assessment of outcome).

After the above exclusions a total of 117 patients were interviewed

and examined by the three treating physicians **(11. G. K.,** T. A. D., B. C. E.), 82 being accepted and 35 rejected. The reasons for rejection were recent exacerbation of chronic pain (3), overt psychopathology (3) and radiographic osteoporosis (1), alcohol abuse (2), cervical myelopathy (I), upper rather than lower back pain (3), uncontrolled diabetes, angina or hypertension (4), aseptic necrosis or osteoarthritis of the hips (2), "total body" pain (2), unresolved litigation (2), other conservative treatment not tried (1), and refusal to participate (11). All patients accepted for the study had full clinical evaluation as well as lumbar spine and pelvic X-rays and laboratory tests to rule out infectious, neoplastic, metabolic, or inflammatory causes of back pain.

The patients had tried a wide range of non-surgical treatments, from chiropractic manipulation to acupuncture and corticosteroid facet injections. At entry into the study 49 (60%) were taking non-steroidal anti-inflammatory drugs and 6 (7%) were taking narcotic analgesics. The most common historical features were a need to change positions after prolonged posture (91.%), avoidance

of lifting heavy weights (70%), difficulty in getting out of a chair (65%), and pain interfering with sleep (65%). Only 17% had to restrict their walking up to 30 min or less and 21% had to decrease their frequency of sexual activity. Nine % of patients stayed at home most of the time because o their back pain and 4% stayed in bed most of the time. Patients were examined neurologically to rule out central and peripheral nervous system disease including acute radiculopathy.

In all patients staight leg raising was possible to at least 70 degrees without pain.

Consent

All eligible patients were informed as to the nature of the study and the possibilities of side effects or complications, including the remote possibility of death or paralysis. The study was approved and monitored by the Sansum Medical Research Foundation Institutional Review Board. Written informed consent was obtained from all patients.

Randomisation

Patients were allocated by the statistician (L. J. H.) into the experimental placebo group by means of a random numbers table. Patients were also randomly assigned to one of the three treating physicians for the double-blind treatment and to a different physician for the manipulation, which of necessity was single blinded.

Statistical Power

To have a power value of 90%, a total of 34 patients would be needed in each group, according to our estimates of an 80% response rate in the experimental group and a 40% response rate in the placebo group. The determination of sample size was based on a simple binomial proportion test to give power with an alpha level level of 0.05. By recruiting 82 patients for the study we allowed sufficient margin for attrition.

Other Treatments

Patients were advised to stop all pain medications except paracetamol (acetaminophen) and to avoid all other ancillary forms of treatment for back pain during the course of the study.

Injected Solutions

The experimental solution consisted of dextrose 25% (694 mosmol/l), glycerine 25% (2720 mosmol/l), phenol 2.5% (266 mosmol/l), and pyrogen-free water to 100%. Because this solution may cause a temporary irritation it was diluted with an equal volume of 0-5% plain lignocaine hydrochloride (`Xylocaine') to make it comparable with the placebo injection in terms of initial provocation of post-injection. Patients in the placebo group received sterile 0-9% saline. Each patient received six injections of approximately 20 ml of the same solution weekly. The solutions were identical in appearance and were prepared by a pharmacist using sterile techniques. Phenol has a characteristic odour that might be detectable if a drop of solution was spilled. This potential source of bias was eliminated by addition of phenol to the skin preparation throughout the study.

Protocol

Differences between experimental and control protocols are outlined in Table I.

Day one.—The study coordinator informed each of the three injecting physicians whether to administer the experimental or placebo treatment to each patient assigned to him for this day only.

All patients were given 10 mg diazepam intravenously for relaxation and amnesia before the start of treatment. Patients in the experimental group were injected with 0-5% lignocaine in the following manner. The spinous process of L5 was identified and the skin overlying this area was sterilised and anaesthetised. A rigid 7-6 cm or 8-9 cm (19-gauge) needle was used for all injections. All injections were made from this single insertion into (1) tip of the spinous process of L4 and L5 and associated supraspinous and interspinous ligaments; (2) attachment of the ligamentum flavurn along the borders of L4 and L5 laminae; (3) apophyseal joint capsules at L4-5, L5- . I; (4) attachment of the iliolumbar ligaments at the transverse process of L4 and L5; (5) attachment of the iliolumbar ligament and dorsolumbar fascia to the iliac crest; and (6) attachments of the short and long fibres of the posterior sacroiliac ligaments, and the sacral and iliac attachments of the interosseous sacroiliac ligaments. Hackett[1] described a characteristic pattern of referred pain from the sacrospinous and sacrotuberous ligaments.

When this pattern was encountered additional injections were made from a separate entry point into the sacrospinous and sacrotuberous ligament origins along the lateral sacral border.

TABLE I—SUMMARY OF TREATMENT PROTOCOL

—	Experimental	Placebo
Day one (single-blind)	1. Infiltration of 60 ml 0·5% lignocaine into specific sites 2. Forceful manipulation 3. Infiltration of triamcinolone into gluteus medius origin	Less than 10 ml 0·5% lignocaine injected at same sites Non-forceful manipulation Infiltration of lignocaine into gluteus medius origin
Day two (double-blind)	1. Injection of proliferant into specific ligamentous and fascial sites 2. Repeated therapeutic flexion exercises	Injection of sterile saline into same sites Same as experimental group
Week 2–6 (double-blind)	Continued exercises and weekly injections of proliferant	Continued exercises and weekly injections of saline

A maximum of 60 ml 0·5% lignocaine was used in the experimental group patients.

The placebo patients were injected at the same entry site(s) with 0·5% lignocaine, but no more than 10 ml was used. Gluteal muscle irritation, which we have found to be a nearly universal phenomenon in chronic back pain patients, was treated in the experimental by infiltration of 50 mg triamcinolone in 10 ml 0·5% lignocaine to the fascial origin primarily of the gluteus medius muscle. placebo patients were injected with lignocaine alone. A forceful manipulation was then performed in the experimental group patients. This was a modified version of the "typical" sacro lumbar roll, The manipulation required an assistant to immobilise the thorax, the thigh being used as a lever to achieve a rotary flexion strain across the sacroiliac and low lumbar areas. Patients in the placebo group received a manipulation in which they were placed on their side and pressure was applied from behind to the torso and buttocks simultaneously. This manoeuvre "rolled" the patient without producing any torsion across the lumbar pine or sacroiliac joints. Patients were amnesic for the procedure owing to the diazepam and were not told that two different forms of manipulation were being used. In no instance did a placebo patient indicate awareness that anything other than a "true" manipulation had been performed.

Subsequent treatment—All subsequent injections were given in double-blind fashion by a physician who had not performed the manipulation. Patients in the experimental group received the first of six weekly injections of 20 ml experimental solution into the same sites as described above for the lignocaine injection, 0.2-0-4 ml being used at each site. Patients in the placebo group were injected with 20 ml ph 'cal saline into these same sites. These injections were r ted weekly for the succeeding five weeks by the same physician in double-blind manner. About 85% of patients in both groups requested and were given premedication with intravenous-diazepam, with or without pethidine, to lessen the discomfort of the weekly injections. Patients in both groups were instructed in a specific series of flexion exercises. These exercises were continued during the injection period and for at least six months afterwards. The primary exercise consisted of standing with feet together and flexing forward at least 150 times daily. The exercises were modified to an easier sitting version in those patients for whom standing flexion proved too painful or vigorous. Although there is a theOretical objection to flexion exercises (increased intradiscal pressure), we have not found them harmful in the context of = present treatment regimen. All patients were repeatedly • to use their backs and to perform previously

painful activity.

Monitoring for Toxicity

During the w*eek after each* injection patients completed a comprehensive questionnaire about subjective complaints. All patients had a complete blood count, sedimentation rate, urinalysis, chemistry panel, and thyroid function tests done before the beginning of the study and after the fourth in the series of six injections. Abnormal values were followed up with repeat tests.

Assessment of Outcome

The success of any treatment for low back pain must rest on the patient's subjective assessment of pain and disability.[10]

Disability and pain scores—We used a previously validated disability questionnaire designed by Roland,[11] consisting of 24 questions. An additional 9 questions were added from Waddell's chronic disability index,[12] making a total of 33. The disability pain score was calculated by adding the number of positive responses out of 33. The emphasis of these questions was on loss of function in the performance of everyday activities rather than on the level of pain. A visual analogue pain scale represented by a straight line scored from a low of 0 cm (no pain) to a high of 7.5 cm (severe pain) was marked by the patient at all visits. Disability and visual analogue pain scores were assessed at baseline and one, three, and six months from completion of treatment. Each patient completed a pain diagram, which was analysed for area of pain by counting the number of grids marked. The maximum number of 102 included all tissue below the mid lumbar spine as well as the lower extremities. An analysis was *made* to identify 'the number of patients in each group with pain radiation into the lower extremity below the knee.

Clinical Signs

The injecting physician was not involved in *the* evaluation. All clinical signs w determined by an independent "blinded" observer who had no other contact with the study patients. (1) A modification" of Schober's technique was used to measure anterior spinal fiction. Three marks were made on the skin with the subject standing erect. The first was at the lumbosacral junction, then 5 cm below and 10 cm above this point. The patient bent forward and the new distance between the upper and lower marks was measured. (2) The examiner's thumbs were placed over the posterior superior iliac spines of the standing or seated patient. The patient bent forward as far as possible and an estimate was made as to whether the upward movement of the thumbs was symmetrical.[9] (3) Patients were examined from behind while standing erect for symmetry of range of motion. If there was a pelvic tilt these tests were performed with the patient seated. (4) Gluteal irritation was said to be present if there was visible asymmetry of movement of the buttock on forward flexion of the lumbar spine and localised spasm or fasiculation coupled with localised tenderness of the fascial origin of the gluteal muscle group.

Breaking of Code and Data Analysis

During the planning of the study the decision was made to observe the patients and analyse their disability and visual analogue scores double-blind for a minimum of six months from completion of treatment, and longer if the groups diverged without reaching statistical significance. All analyses including the calculation of Pearson correlation coefficients for the subjective and clinical data were performed by SYSTAT implemented on an IBM PC; AT.

Statistical tests were based upon simple independent and dependent tests for continuous variables, and in those instances in which a variable was dichotomised, the Yates corrected chi-square was used.

Results

After randomisation 42 patients were in the placebo group and 40 in the experimental group. One patient in the placebo group dropped out, leaving 81 for evaluation during the six months of double-blind follow-up. The two groups were clinically similar at entry (Table II).

Subjective Scores

One month after treatment both groups had improved in terms of disability and visual analogue pain scores, but the improvement was significantly greater in the experimental group at this time and at three and six months (Table III). Thirty-five of 40 patients in the experimental group had greater than 50% improvement in disability scores, compared with 16 of 41 in the control group; and the numbers with zero disability scores at six months were 15 and 4, respectively (p < 0·003).

The pain diagram grid score likewise showed changes favouring the experimental treatment (Table III). At the onset of the study 12 patients in the experimental group and 12 in the placebo group had pain radiating into the distal part of one or both legs. At six months this had resolved completely in 10 and 2, respectively (p < 0·01).

Clinical signs

Independent evaluation of physical signs revealed no significant differences between the groups after treatment.

We tested the Pearson correlation irrespective of treatment group between all subjective and "objective" data recorded in the study.

TABLE II—COMPARABILITY OF PATIENTS AT BASELINE

—	Experimental (n = 40)	Placebo (n = 41)
Mean age, SEM (range)	45, 2·08 (23–70)	43·3, 1·66 (23–70)
M/F	18/22	20/21
Years of pain:		
mean, SEM (range)	8·98, 1·03 (1–30)	10·72, 1·38 (1–35)
X-ray findings:		
Normal	11	12
Disc narrowing	6	12
Degen changes	3	2
Disc and degen changes	20	15
Disability score (33 maximum) mean, SEM (range)	11·45, 0·83 (4–26)	11·83, 0·91 (4–26)
Visual analogue pain score (7·5 maximum) mean, SEM (range)	3·76, 0·19 (1·5–7·2)	4·0, 0·18 (1·2–6·0)
Pain grid score (102 maximum) mean, SEM (range)	10·1, 1·24 (1–38)	10·27, 1·6 (2–33)
No of patients with radiation of pain into distal lower extremity	12	12

TABLE III—SUBJECTIVE SCORES*

—	Placebo	Experimental	p
Disability			
Entry	11·82 (0·92)	11·45 (0·83)	—
1 mo	8·37 (1·04)	4·00 (0·61)	<0·001
3 mo	8·49 (1·04)	4·70 (0·73)	<0·004
6 mo	8·29 (1·10)	3·43 (0·72)	<0·001
Pain (visual analogue)			
Entry	3·99 (0·19)	3·78 (0·19)	—
1 mo	3·06 (0·29)	2·13 (0·22)	<0·01
3 mo	2·93 (0·25)	1·77 (0·22)	<0·001
6 mo	3·08 (0·28)	1·50 (0·21)	<0·001
Pain (grid)			
Entry	10·27 (1·6)	10·1 (1·24)	
6 mo	8·24 (1·20)	3·6 (0·37)	<0·001

*Mean (SEM).

Only two physical findings showed a correlation (p <0·05) with the visual analogue pain score at six months—namely, the return of rotational symmetry (r = 0.315) and the absence of gluteal irritation (r = 0·271).

Side-effects and Laboratory Data

Patients in both groups complained of pain and stiffness for 12-24 h after each injection; this was never severe enough to necessitate bed rest or absence from work. 2 *patients* in the experimental group and 1 in the control group had an increase in menstrual flow and 2 in the experimental group had postmenopausal spotting four weeks after starting treatment. One patient in the placebo group withdrew after the day-two injections because of severe headache and cough; these had resolved at follow-up a week later. There were no significant differences in laboratory data from the two groups.

DISCUSSION

The sacroiliac joint has a small range of motion, and when the joint is at the limit of its range no great force is needed to damage its ligaments.[14] Once the ligaments of the low back and pelvis become incompetent, instability results.

This permits excessive external moments to be transmitted to the three-joint complex of intervertebral disc and zygapophyseal joints,[15] and torsional stresses to be placed on the lumbar vertebrae and sacrum. The former may lead to disc and zygapophyseal joint degeneration and the latter to a slight displacement of the sacrum from its normal anatomic position,[14] placing traction on pain sensitive structures and producing local as well as referred pain.

The treatment programme tested here has multiple components. We offer the following speculations as to why it is effective. The lute lignocaine serves to interrupt the pain reflex arc and facilitate the manipulation. Triamcinolone "disinflames" the gluteal muscles, which are subjected to chronic mechanical strain owing to the incompetence of the lumbar and sacroiliac ligaments. The manipulation moves the sacroiliac joint through a full range of motion, rupturing any microadhesions which may form in response to connective tissue immobilisation,[16] and corrects any minor sacral malalignment present. The transient benefits previously demonstrated with manipulation[17] are usually not sustained less the supporting ligaments are strengthened. The proliferant induces an inflammatory response which leads to fibroblastic hyperplasia and the growth of collagen.[1] The exercises encourage synthesis of the extracellular connective tissue matnx,[16] increase ligament junction strength,[18] and induce proliferating fibroblasts to line up in parallel to existing connective tissue.[19]

In designing the protocol for the study we were faced with the dilemma of testing each component of the system in order to isolate its relative contribution, or testing the system as a whole. The repeated needling is painful, and it is a tribute to the study participants and a commentary on the desperate plight of patients with chronic pain that only patient dropped out. We were unable logistically to justify treating a larger number of patients. We therefore elected to compare the complete system of treatment with a parallel but placebo system. Future studies may be needed to analyse the relative import of each component of the overall procedure. We conclude that the experimental regimen is a safe and effective treatment for chronic low back pain that has not responded to other conservative forms of treatment.

We thank Lynne Cantlay, PH D, for organisational help; the nursing staff of the Sansum Clinic. and especially Ms Alice Dalton, for skilled assistance; William Kubitschek, DO, for helpful suggestions; Charles Peterson, MD, for assistance in evaluating clinical signs; W. H. Kirkaldy-Willis, MD, for review of the script; Steve Cooley, PHARM D for preparing the injectable solutions; Ms Rose Louie for serving as study coordinator; Sid Mauk, MD, for interpretation Of radiographs; and Carl Johnson, MD, for evaluating the biopsy specimens.

Correspondence should be addressed to R. G. K.,

Sansum Medical Clinic
317 W. Pueblo. PO Drawer LL
Santa Barbara, CA 93102,
USA.

REFERENCES

1. Hackett GS. Ligament and tendon relaxation treated by prolotherapy, 3rd ed.
Springfield: Clarks C Thomas, 1958.

"P. Copiais C. T. Th. conservative treatment of low back pain. In: Helfet A J, Gruebel Lee DM, eds. Disorders of the lumbar spine. Philadelphia: Lippincott, 1978: 145-83.

3. Peterson TM, Injection treatment for back pain. *Am j Orthop* 1963; 5: 320-25.

4. Myers A. Proiotherapy treatment of low back pain and *sciatica. Bull Hasp joint Dis* 1961; 22: 48-55.

5. Neff F. Back pain and disability. if' *Med* 1960; 1: 12-17.

6. Hunt WE, Baird WC. Complications following injections of sclerosing agent to precipitate fibro-osseous proliferation. *J Neurosurg* 1961; 18: 461-65.

7. Keptinger JE, Bucy PC. Paraplegia from treatment with sclerosing agents---report of a case. PIMA 1960; 73: 1333-36.

8. Schneider RC. Williams J1, Liss L. Fatality after injection of sclerosing agent to precipitate fibro-osseous proliferation. 'AMA 1959; 170: 1768-72.

9. Bourdilbon JF. Spinal manipulation, 3rd ed. New York: Appleton-Century Crafts. 1982: 49-122.

10. Million R, Hall W, Haavik Nilsen K, Baker RD, Jayson M1V. Assessment of the progress of the back pain patient. Spine 1982; 7: 204-12.

11. Roland MR, Morris RM. A study of the natural history of low back pain. Spate 1983; 145-50.

12. Waddell G. Main CI. Assessment of seventy in low back disorders. Spine 1984; 9:204-013.

13. Merritt JL, McLean TI, Erickson RP, Offord KP. Measurement of trunk flexibility in normal subjects: reproducibility of three clinical methods. Mayo Clin Proc 1986:61: 192-97.

14. Grieve EFM. Mechanical dysfunction of the sacroiliac joint. Int Rehab Med 1983; 5:46-52.

15. Kirkaldy-Willis WH, ed. The pathology and pathogenesis of low back pain. In: Managing low back pain. New York: Churchill Livingstone, 1983: 23-44.

16. Nimni M. Collagen: Structure, function, and metabolism in normal and fibrotic tissues. Sem Arch Rheum 1983; 13: 1-86.

17. Radler NM. Diagnosis and treatment of backache. In: Medical management of the regional musculoskeletal diseases. Orlando: Grune and Stratton, 1984: 3-52.

18. Tipton CM, Marthes RD, Sandage DS. In situ measurement of junction strength and ligament elongation in rats. J Appl Phytiol 1974; 37: 758-61.

19. Bunting CH, Eades CC. The effect of mechanical tension upon the polarity of growing fibroblasts. Exp Med 1926; 44: 147-49.

Chapter Seven

LIGAMENT INSTABILITY OF KNEES

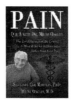

Ligament instability of knees: a new approach to treatment

Milne J. Ongley, Thomas A. Dorman, Bjorn C. Eek, David Lundgren, and Robert G. Klein.

Costa Mesa, California, USA

Summary. Prolotherapy was shown to be effective for ligament strengthening in five injured knees, measured by objective instrumentation.

Key words: Knee—Prolotherapy—Sclerotherapy—Ligament —Ligament strength measurement.

Injuries to the knee can result in ligamentous instability with resultant pain. Standard surgical treatment is to immobilize the knee and if pain and instability continue, surgical intervention may be necessary. However, surgical reconstruction has resulted in varying success [2, 3, 5, 6] and therefore the best approach remains controversial.

We have developed a new treatment using proliferant injection therapy into the ligament to provide sclerosis and tightening of the ligaments.

Proliferant injection therapy is based on the principle hypotheses that: (1) interstitial rupture of collagen fibers within the substance of ligaments produces elongation and thus dysfunction; (2) repeated provocation of an inflammatory reaction within the ligament will induce fibroblastic hyperplasia and the laying down of new collagen; hence (3) ligament healing may be achieved in the presence of normal active movement.

In the knee proliferant injection has not hitherto been subject to critical analysis in a clinical setting.

The popularity of sclerosing injections into ligaments for the relief of instability and pain has fluctuated since the late 1950s due to the side effect of the solutions in vogue at that time, i.e. severe pain production, which often required hospitalization and narcotics.

With a new proliferant solution we studied the response to multiple injections into the posterior, anterior cruciate and the medial and lateral collateral ligaments.

Materials and methods

Patients

The study was conducted during a 9-month period in a private orthopedic office. Thirty patients presented with knee pain during the enrollment period, but five knees (in four patients) were selected because of substantial and reproducible ligament instability. After informed consent had been given specific measurements were obtained.

Offprint requests to: Th. A. Dorman, 1041, Murray Avenue, San Luis

Obispo, California, 93401, USA

All measurements were taken by one researcher (D. L.). The patients underwent multiple injections and were followed routinely. After 9 months repeated measurements were obtained. Subjective symptoms were recorded at entry and exit from the study.

Measurements

Ligament stability was measured by a commercially available computerized instrument that measures ligament function objectively and reliably in a complete three-dimensional format 17, 91. It consists of a chair equipped with a six-component force platform and a 6' freedom electrogoniometer. With computer-integrated force and motion measurements, a standardized series of clinical laxity tests can be performed and an objective report obtained. Prior studies have compared clinical testing with objective tests Ill and have established reproducibility 14).

Proliferant solution

The proliferant solution is made up as follows: dextrose 25% (694mosmoi/i), glycerine 25% (2720mosmoi/i), phenol 2.5% (266-mosmottl), and pyrogen-free water to 100%. At the time of injection it is diluted with an equal volume of 0.5% lidocaine.

The proliferant injections are "peppered" into the lax ligament(s) usually at 2-weekly intervals, each offending ligament being treated an average of four times. A total of between 30 and 40cc of the proliferant solution is injected into the appropriate portion of the joint ligaments.

Intervention—Injection

The posterior cruciate ligament. Each end is injected from a separate needle insertion site. The anterior end is approached with the patient supine and with the lower limb extended. The superior attachment is masked by the patella; therefore it is necessary for the surgeon to tilt the patella from the femoral condyle in a medial direction. A 19-gauge 3" needle is inserted at the lateral patellar margin and travels medially parallel to the articular surfaces. When the needle hits the lateral aspect of the medial femoral condyle, its position is adjusted until ligamentous resistance is felt. The injection is made by a series of tiny withdrawals and reinsertions, injecting 0.1 cc at a time until the insertion is thoroughly peppered.

The needle is then "walked" down the ligament as far as possible, peppering the body of the ligament.

Treatment of the posterior end of the posterior cruciate ligament is accomplished with the patient prone and the knee very Slightly flexed. For this approach it is essential to bypass he popliteal vessels which overlie the posterior attachment. An easy approach is to employ one's thumb to locate the apex of the lateral condyle. The needle is inserted there and is inclined at about 60° to the horizontal. It thus passes well under the popliteal vessels and heads distally towards the center of the posterior aspect of the tibia. The angle of entry is then progressively altered until the needle is felt to penetrate the ligament.

A series of small injections is made, 0.1 cc at a time, until the insertion of the ligament is thoroughly peppered; the needle is then walked up the ligament, peppering it with the proliferant solution as far as possible.

The anterior cruciate ligament. The anterior end is approached with the patient supine and the knee flexed to 90°. The needle enters immediately below the medial edge of the patella at an angle of about 45°. It is aimed for the spine of the tibia; the tip penetrates a resilient tissue—the ligament—before striking bone. The infiltration is made as before by a series of tiny withdrawals and reinsertions, as previously described, until the attachment is thoroughly peppered.

The treatment of the *posterior end* mirrors the method used for the posterior end of the posterior cruciate, in that the popliteal vessels must be negotiated. The approach is from the medial side, pointing slightly proximally. This time the apex of the medial condyle is identified and the needle punctures the skin at an angle about half way between vertical and horizontal. The tip is directed towards the medial surface of the lateral condyle and the ligamentous resistance is encountered before hitting bone. The injection is made by a series of withdrawals and reinsertions 0.1 cc at a time, thoroughly peppering the ligament insertion and as much of the ligament as possible by walking the needle up the ligament.

The lateral collateral ligament is identified by palpation and infiltrated from an insertion point about 4 cm anterior to it so that the peppering technique can allow the operator to infiltrate it along the whole of its length, paying particular attention to its insertions.

The medial collateral ligament is more intimately attached to the capsule and broader than the lateral one, but the method of injection is analogous.

Table 1. Objective and subjective data (all measurements in mm)

Pt.	90°/0° Flx/Rtn		90°/10°IR Flx/Rtn		30°/0° Flx/Rtn		80° Int/ext Rtn. stress in deg.		Areas treated	Subjective before treatment	Subjective after 9 months follow up
Rx	before	after	before	after	before	after	before	after			
DT 27M L	10	6	6	3	12	5	38	33	MCL; LCL; PCL; ACL Med/lat caps	Pain; instability; unable to run, play tennis; feels insecure with weight bearing; Left medial menisectomy 1982	No pain, more stable; able to run; starting to play tennis + less aware of knees
R	9	8	6	3	20	13	47	36	MCL; LCL; PCL; ACL Med/lat caps	Right partial menisectomy 1984	
GS 35M R	13	8	8	4	10	7	37	37	MCL; LCL; ACL; PCL Med caps	sprained R knee skiing March 1986; knee unstable; weak; unable to bicycle	More stable; able to bicycle 30 – 40 miles
SW 31F R	7	5	7	1	5	2	54	41	MCL; LCL; PCL; Med/lat/ant caps	Right medial menisectomy 1971; pain and instability with activities; minimal activity level	No pain; more stable; moderate to marked level of activities; able to cycle/W. Ski
KW 43F R	8	4	7	3	5	0	40	31	MCL; LCL; PCL; Ant/post Med/lat caps	Right knee pain since February 1985 when she fell, causing fracture/dislocation of right angle; pain, weakness and instability	Decrease in pain; more stable; tolerating increase in activity and starting resistive exercises
P value	0.013	0.002	0.005	0.03							

MCL = medial collateral ligament; LCL = lateral collateral ligament; PCL = posterior cruciate ligament; ACL = anterior cruciate ligament; Caps = capsule

The injection is immediately followed by low-resistance ergor-netric bicycle exercise for half an hour. This exercise is repeated at least daily in the interval between office visits. Experience has shown that this exercise reduces or abolishes painful reactions and large effusions in the treated knees.

Results

Table I illustrates the measurements of the five knees in the three-dimensional computerized format.

The tests performed were: (1) 90° antero-posteriorcaine (A-P) draw; 2 90° A -P draw with internal rotation of

10°; (3) 30° A-P draw (Lachman); (4) 80° internal-external rotation stress.

In the 90°/0° internal rotation A-P draw the range of displacement was 7-13 mm (mean = 9.4, SD = 2.059) before the intervention. After proliferant therapy with physiotherapy the range in the A-P draw was 4-8 mm (mean = 6.2, SD = 1.6), Using the t -test for pre-post treatment, the P value was 0.013.

In the 90°/100 internal rotation A-P draw the range of displacement was 6-8mm (mean=6.8, SD=0.748) before the intervention. After proliferant therapy with physiotherapy the range in the same test was 1 - 4 mm (mean = 2.8, SD = 0.979). Using the 1-test for pre-post treatment, the P value was 0.002.

In the 30°/0° (Lachman) A -P draw the range of displacement was 5-20 mm (mean = 10.4, SD = 5.535) before the intervention. After proliferant therapy with physiotherapy the range in the A-P draw was 0-1 3 mm (mean = 5.4, '41) 4.499). Using the t-test for pre-post treatment, *the* P value was 0.005.

In the 80°/0" internal external rotation stress in degrees the range of displacement was 38"-47° (mean = 4:1.2, SD = 6.431) before the intervention. After proliferant therapy with physiotherapy the range in the same test was 31°-37° (mean = 35.6, SD = 3.440). Using the t-test for pre-post treatment, the P value was 0.03.

All demonstrate statistical significance at P<0.05. The subjective changes are listed on the right-hand side of Table I The most impressive changes were in reduction of pain in all subjects with an increase in activities as listed In Table 1.

Complications and side effects

No systemic or general complications occurred in the four eases who comprise the population of this report, or any of the other patients, who were not available for retesting on the Genucom.

In a number of cases an effusion and swelling develops after a proliferant injection by this therapeutic method. The five knees which are the basis of this report were managed expectantly, there being minimal or no local reactions. In some other instances, however, triamcinolone suspension (40 mg) with local anesthesia (lidocaine 0.5%) as a vehicle, is used when there is an acute inflammation from an injury, or to "cool down" a joint from an excessive inflammatory reaction induced by proliferant therapy.

Subsequently, the treatment routine is resumed, and the end result is no less satisfactory.

Discussion

We interpret these data to indicate that our protocol was successful in reducing the laxity of unstable knees in our study group. All patients demonstrated improvement in measurable objective data. In addition, the subjective improvement and activity level was markedly improved.

This study is one of the first to measure clinical outcome by the three-dimensional computerized instrument. We believe this technique will help to evaluate intervention in unstable knees. The technique was practical and could easily be adapted for routine clinical work. The prolotherapy provided a well-tolerated new dimension in the treatment of ligamentous instability of the knee. It was well tolerated, as the preliminary results demonstrated. In other studies of proliferant therapy [8] excellent results have previously been reported.

The study limitations are the small number of subjects and the study design. A randomized control without injection therapy and only physiotherapy will be necessary to confirm bur results. We believe, however, that our results are very encouraging and provide the scientific format for further research.

Acknowledgements.

We wish to thank FARO Medical Technologies Inc., 2875 Sabourin, Montreal, Quebec, Canada, H4S 1M9 for providing the Genacom computerized instrument during the study, and Lawrence J. Hubert Ph. D. for the statistical analysis.

References

1. Daniel DM, Malcolm Li., Losse o, Stone ML, Sachs R, Burks R (1985) Instrument measurement of anterior laxity of the knee. J Bone Joint burg [Am] 67:720-725.

2. Fried JA, Berfield JA, Weiker G, Andrish JT (1985) Anterior eructate reconstruction using the Jones-Ellison procedure. J Bone Joint Surg [Am] 67:1029-- 1033

3. Haughston IC, Jacobson KE (1985) Chronic posterolateral rotary instability of the knee. J Bone Joint Surg [AM]

67:351-359

4. Highgenboteh CL (1980) The reliability of the Genucom knee analysis system, The Second European Congress of Knee Surgery ans Arthrbscopy held in Basle, Switzerland, September 29

5. Insall JN (1984] Surgery of the knee. Chronic instability of the knee. Churchill Livingstone, New York, p 295

6. Neugebauer R, Burri C (1985) Carbon fiber ligament replacement in chronic knee Instability. Clin Orthop 196:118-123

7. Oliver JH, Coughlin LP (1985) An analysis of knee evaluation using clinical techniques and the Genucom knee analysis system. American Orthopedic Society for Sports Medicine, Interim Meeting, January 23-24, Las Vegas, Nevada

8. Ongley MJ, Klein RG, Dorman TA, Eek BC, Hubert L (1987) A new approach to the treatment of chronic low-back pain. Lancet II: 143-146

9. Selsnick H, Oliver J, Virgin C (1986) Analysis o f knee ligament testing-Getimicom and clinical exams. American Orthopedic
Society of Sports Medicine, Annual Meeting, Sun Valley, Idaho, July
14-17

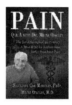

- NCBI
  - Skip to main content
  - Skip to navigation
  - Resources
  - All Resources
  - Chemicals & Bioassays
    - BioSystems
    - PubChem BioAssay
    - PubChem Compound
    - PubChem Structure Search
    - PubChem Substance
    - All Chemicals & Bioassays Resources...
  - DNA & RNA
    - BLAST (Basic Local Alignment Search Tool)
    - BLAST (Stand-alone)
    - E-Utilities
    - GenBank
    - GenBank: BankIt
    - GenBank: Sequin

- GenBank: tbl2asn
- Genome Workbench
- Influenza Virus
- Nucleotide Database
- PopSet
- Primer-BLAST
- ProSplign
- Reference Sequence (RefSeq)
- RefSeqGene
- Sequence Read Archive (SRA)
- Splign
- Trace Archive
- All DNA & RNA Resources...
○ Data & Software
- BLAST (Basic Local Alignment Search Tool)
- BLAST (Stand-alone)
- Cn3D
- Conserved Domain Search Service (CD Search)
- E-Utilities
- GenBank: BankIt
- GenBank: Sequin
- GenBank: tbl2asn
- Genome ProtMap
- Genome Workbench
- Primer-BLAST
- ProSplign
- PubChem Structure Search
- SNP Submission Tool
- Splign
- Vector Alignment Search Tool (VAST)
- All Data & Software Resources...
○ Domains & Structures
- BioSystems
- Cn3D

- Conserved Domain Database (CDD)
- Conserved Domain Search Service (CD Search)
- Structure (Molecular Modeling Database)
- Vector Alignment Search Tool (VAST)
- All Domains & Structures Resources...
○ Genes & Expression
- BioSystems
- Database of Genotypes and Phenotypes (dbGaP)
- E-Utilities
- Gene
- Gene Expression Omnibus (GEO) Database
- Gene Expression Omnibus (GEO) Datasets
- Gene Expression Omnibus (GEO) Profiles
- Genome Workbench
- HomoloGene
- Online Mendelian Inheritance in Man (OMIM)
- RefSeqGene
- All Genes & Expression Resources...
○ Genetics & Medicine
- Bookshelf
- Database of Genotypes and Phenotypes (dbGaP)
- Genetic Testing Registry
- Influenza Virus
- Online Mendelian Inheritance in Man (OMIM)
- PubMed
- PubMed Central (PMC)
- PubMed Clinical Queries
- RefSeqGene
- All Genetics & Medicine Resources...
○ Genomes & Maps
- Database of Genomic Structural Variation (dbVar)
- GenBank: tbl2asn
- Genome
- Genome Project

- Genome Data Viewer (GDV)
- Genome ProtMap
- Genome Workbench
- Influenza Virus
- Nucleotide Database
- PopSet
- ProSplign
- Sequence Read Archive (SRA)
- Splign
- Trace Archive
- All Genomes & Maps Resources...
◦ Homology
- BLAST (Basic Local Alignment Search Tool)
- BLAST (Stand-alone)
- BLAST Link (BLink)
- Conserved Domain Database (CDD)
- Conserved Domain Search Service (CD Search)
- Genome ProtMap
- HomoloGene
- Protein Clusters
- All Homology Resources...
◦ Literature
- Bookshelf
- E-Utilities
- Journals in NCBI Databases
- MeSH Database
- NCBI Handbook
- NCBI Help Manual
- NCBI News & Blog
- PubMed
- PubMed Central (PMC)
- PubMed Clinical Queries
- All Literature Resources...
◦ Proteins

- BioSystems
- BLAST (Basic Local Alignment Search Tool)
- BLAST (Stand-alone)
- BLAST Link (BLink)
- Conserved Domain Database (CDD)
- Conserved Domain Search Service (CD Search)
- E-Utilities
- ProSplign
- Protein Clusters
- Protein Database
- Reference Sequence (RefSeq)
- All Proteins Resources...
○ Sequence Analysis
- BLAST (Basic Local Alignment Search Tool)
- BLAST (Stand-alone)
- BLAST Link (BLink)
- Conserved Domain Search Service (CD Search)
- Genome ProtMap
- Genome Workbench
- Influenza Virus
- Primer-BLAST
- ProSplign
- Splign
- All Sequence Analysis Resources...
○ Taxonomy
- Taxonomy
- Taxonomy Browser
- Taxonomy Common Tree
- All Taxonomy Resources...
○ Training & Tutorials
- NCBI Education Page
- NCBI Handbook
- NCBI Help Manual
- NCBI News & Blog

- All Training & Tutorials Resources...
○ Variation
- Database of Genomic Structural Variation (dbVar)
- Database of Genotypes and Phenotypes (dbGaP)
- Database of Single Nucleotide Polymorphisms (dbSNP)
- SNP Submission Tool
- All Variation Resources...
• How To
○ All How To
○ Chemicals & Bioassays
○ DNA & RNA
○ Data & Software
○ Domains & Structures
○ Genes & Expression
○ Genetics & Medicine
○ Genomes & Maps
○ Homology
○ Literature
○ Proteins
○ Sequence Analysis
○ Taxonomy
○ Training & Tutorials
○ Variation
• About NCBI Accesskeys
drdphdMy NCBISign Out

PubMed

US National Library of Medicine National Institutes of Health
Search databasePubMedBooksAll DatabasesAssemblyBiocol-
lectionsBioProjectBioSampleBioSystemsBooksClinVarConserved
DomainsdbGaPdbVarGeneGenomeGEO   DataSetsGEO
ProfilesGTRHomoloGeneIdentical Protein GroupsMedGenMe-
SHNCBI Web SiteNLM CatalogNucleotideOMIMPMCPop-
SetProbeProteinProtein ClustersPubChem BioAssayPubChem

CompoundPubChem   SubstancePubMedSNPSparcleSRAStruc-
tureTaxonomyToolKitToolKitAllToolKitBookgh
   Search term

Search
   • Advanced
   • Help

• Format: Summary
   • Sort by: Best Match
   • Per page: 20
   Send to

Clipboard
   Items: 21 to 30 of 30
   Remove all items
   << First< Prev
   Page 2 of 2
   Next >Last >>

Select item 2354759021.
   Management of chronic tendon injuries.
   Childress MA, Beutler A.
   Am Fam Physician. 2013 Apr 1;87(7):486-90. Review.
   PMID:
   23547590
   Free Article
   Similar articles Remove from clipboard
   Select item 2170358522.

Prolotherapy: a clinical review of its role in treating chronic musculoskeletal pain.

Distel LM, Best TM.

PM R. 2011 Jun;3(6 Suppl 1):S78-81. doi: 10.1016/j.pmrj.2011.04.003. Review.

PMID:

21703585

Similar articles Remove from clipboard

Select item 2018899823.

Prolotherapy in primary care practice.

Rabago D, Slattengren A, Zgierska A.

Prim Care. 2010 Mar;37(1):65-80. doi: 10.1016/j.pop.2009.09.013. Review.

PMID:

20188998

Free PMC Article

Similar articles Remove from clipboard

Select item 1744353724.

Prolotherapy injections for chronic low-back pain.

Dagenais S, Yelland MJ, Del Mar C, Schoene ML.

Cochrane Database Syst Rev. 2007 Apr 18;(2):CD004059. Review.

PMID:

17443537

Similar articles Remove from clipboard

Select item 1635346925.

Prolotherapy (proliferation therapy) in the treatment of TMD.

Hakala RV.

Cranio. 2005 Oct;23(4):283-8. Review.

PMID:

16353469

Similar articles Remove from clipboard

Select item 1616298326.

A systematic review of prolotherapy for chronic musculoskeletal pain.

Rabago D, Best TM, Beamsley M, Patterson J.

Clin J Sport Med. 2005 Sep;15(5):376-80. Review.

PMID:

16162983

Similar articles Remove from clipboard

Select item 1545470327.

Prolotherapy injections for chronic low back pain: a systematic review.

Yelland MJ, Del Mar C, Pirozzo S, Schoene ML.

Spine (Phila Pa 1976). 2004 Oct 1;29(19):2126-33. Review.

PMID:

15454703

Similar articles Remove from clipboard

Select item 1510623428.

Prolotherapy injections for chronic low-back pain.

Yelland MJ, Mar C, Pirozzo S, Schoene ML, Vercoe P.

Cochrane Database Syst Rev. 2004;(2):CD004059. Review. Update in: Cochrane Database Syst Rev. 2007;(2):CD004059.

PMID:

15106234

Similar articles Remove from clipboard

Select item 1510062929.

Critical review of prolotherapy for osteoarthritis, low back pain, and other musculoskeletal conditions: a physiatric perspective.

Kim SR, Stitik TP, Foye PM, Greenwald BD, Campagnolo DI.

Am J Phys Med Rehabil. 2004 May;83(5):379-89. Review.

PMID:

15100629

Similar articles Remove from clipboard

Select item 1458918230.

Prolotherapy at the fringe of medical care, or is it the frontier?

Mooney V.

Spine J. 2003 Jul-Aug;3(4):253-4. Review. No abstract available.
PMID:

14589182

Similar articles Remove from clipboard

<< First< Prev

Page 2 of 2

Next >Last >>

Supplemental Content

Clipboard: 30 items

Filters: Manage Filters

Sort by:

• Best match

• Most recent

Find related data

• Database: SelectAssemblyBioProjectBioSampleBioSystemsBooks-
ClinVarConserved DomainsdbGaPdbVarGeneGenomeGEO Data-
SetsGEO
ProfilesHomoloGeneMedGenNucleotideOMIMPMCPopSet-
ProbeProteinProtein   ClustersPubChem   BioAssayPubChem
CompoundPubChem   SubstancePubMedSNPSRAStructure-
Taxonomy

•

Find items

Recent Activity

ClearTurn OffTurn On

• prolotherapy review AND Review[ptyp] (71)PubMed

· · ·

• Second Chances.PubMed

• Using Preferences - My NCBI Help

• prolotherapy AND (Review[ptyp]) (70)PubMed

• prolotherapy (215)PubMed

Your browsing activity is empty.
    Activity recording is turned off.
    Turn recording back on
    See more...

You are here: NCBI > Literature > PubMed
    Support Center
    Simple NCBI Directory
    • Getting Started

• NCBI Education
    • NCBI Help Manual
    • NCBI Handbook
    • Training & Tutorials
    • Submit Data
    • Resources

• Chemicals & Bioassays
    • Data & Software

- DNA & RNA
- Domains & Structures
- Genes & Expression
- Genetics & Medicine
- Genomes & Maps
- Homology
- Literature
- Proteins
- Sequence Analysis
- Taxonomy
- Variation
- **Popular**

- PubMed
  - Bookshelf
  - PubMed Central
  - BLAST
  - Nucleotide
  - Genome
  - SNP
  - Gene
  - Protein
  - PubChem
  - **Featured**

- Genetic Testing Registry
  - GenBank
  - Reference Sequences
  - Gene Expression Omnibus
  - Genome Data Viewer
  - Human Genome
  - Mouse Genome

- Influenza Virus
- Primer-BLAST
- Sequence Read Archive
- **NCBI Information**

- About NCBI
  - Research at NCBI
  - NCBI News & Blog
  - NCBI FTP Site
  - NCBI on Facebook
  - NCBI on Twitter
  - NCBI on YouTube
  - Privacy Policy
  NLM
  NIH
  DHHS
  USA.gov
  National Center for Biotechnology Information, U.S. National Library of Medicine 8600 Rockville Pike, Bethesda MD, 20894 USA
  Policies and Guidelines | Contact

AFTERWORD

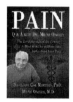

I can say with certainty that meeting Dr. Milne J. Ongley has changed my life. Our conversation shared in the pages of this book encompassed thoughts, emotions, and pain, although Ongley's expertise extends far beyond these topics. He is a man beyond his time, beyond the twenty-first century. I am grateful to you, Dr. Ongley, for sharing some information with us and for being such a dear friend.

It is my hope that in reading his words, you begin to think about life, the human body, and health a little differently. We're all in control of our well-being, and it's up to us to be our own advocate for physical health. If anyone deserves a Noble Prize, it may well be Dr. Ongley, with his foresight and the knowledge of one of the greatest physicians in the twenty-first century.

Now that you've read the insights and glimpsed Dr. Ongley's knowledge, what will you do to improve your physical well-being?

Sieglinde Coe Martens, Ph.D.

Made in the USA
San Bernardino, CA
29 November 2019